GOD DID IT
A True Story of Miraculous Healing

Dianna Hobbs

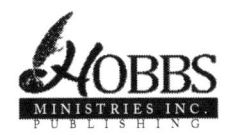

HOBBS MINISTRIES INC.
PUBLISHING

Most Hobbs Ministries book products are available at special quantity discounts for bulk purchase, for sales promotions, premiums, fund-raising, and educational needs. For details, write Empowering Everyday Women Ministries, Inc., 2316 Delaware Ave., #134, Buffalo, NY, 14216.

GOD DID IT by Dianna Hobbs
Published by Hobbs Ministries, Inc.
Hobbs Ministries Publishing/Empowering Everyday Women, Inc.
2316 Delaware Ave.
#134
Buffalo, NY 14216
www.empoweringeverydaywomen.com

All rights reserved. No part of this publication may be reproduced, distributed, or transmitted in any form or by any means, including photocopying, recording, or other electronic or mechanical methods, without the prior written permission of the publisher, except in the case of brief quotations embodied in critical reviews and certain other noncommercial uses permitted by copyright law.

Unless otherwise indicated, all Scripture quotations are from the Holy Bible, New International Version. Copyright © 1973, 1978, 1984, International Bible Society. Used by permission.

Scripture quotations marked NKJV are from the New King James Version of the Bible. Copyright © 1979, 1980, 1982, by Thomas Nelson, Inc. Used by permission.

Scripture quotations marked CEV are from the Contemporary English Version® of the Bible. Copyright © 1995 American Bible Society. Used by permission.

Cover design by Hobbs Ministries/Interior Design by Godzchild publications
Design Director: Ryan Phillips

Copyright © 2018 by Dianna Hobbs
All rights reserved

Printed in the United States of America
First Printing, 2018
ISBN 978-0-692-08986-6

Visit the author's website at www.diannahobbs.com.

TABLE OF CONTENTS

ACKNOWLEDGEMENTS..v

FOREWORD..vii

PREFACE..xix

INTRODUCTION..xxv

PHASE ONE
Covering Up... 1

PHASE TWO
Over It.. 27

PHASE THREE
Asking Why.. 51

PHASE FOUR
Selfishness.. 71

PHASE FIVE
Defeated.. 97

PHASE SIX
Conflicted.. 125

PHASE SEVEN
Healed... 145

ACKNOWLEDGEMENTS

To the God who healed me, I will never cease to praise You. To everyone who prayed for me, thank you.

To the 50 women who interceded for me on March 26, 2017, may God reward you for your selfless service and your commitment to the ministry of intercession.

To everyone who offered support and love, you will never know how much I appreciate you. The fact that you extended yourself in any way, though you didn't have to, will forever be etched in my memory. May the seeds and prayers you all have sown into my life cause a harvest to spring up in yours.

To every doctor, nurse and healthcare worker that went the extra mile to make the going a little easier, I am grateful.

To my loving husband Kenya and our four wonderful children, Kyla, Kaiah, Kedar and Kaleb, thank you for your patience, generosity, encouragement, and for never making me feel like a burden. I love you. Look what the Lord has done. He heard and answered our prayers!

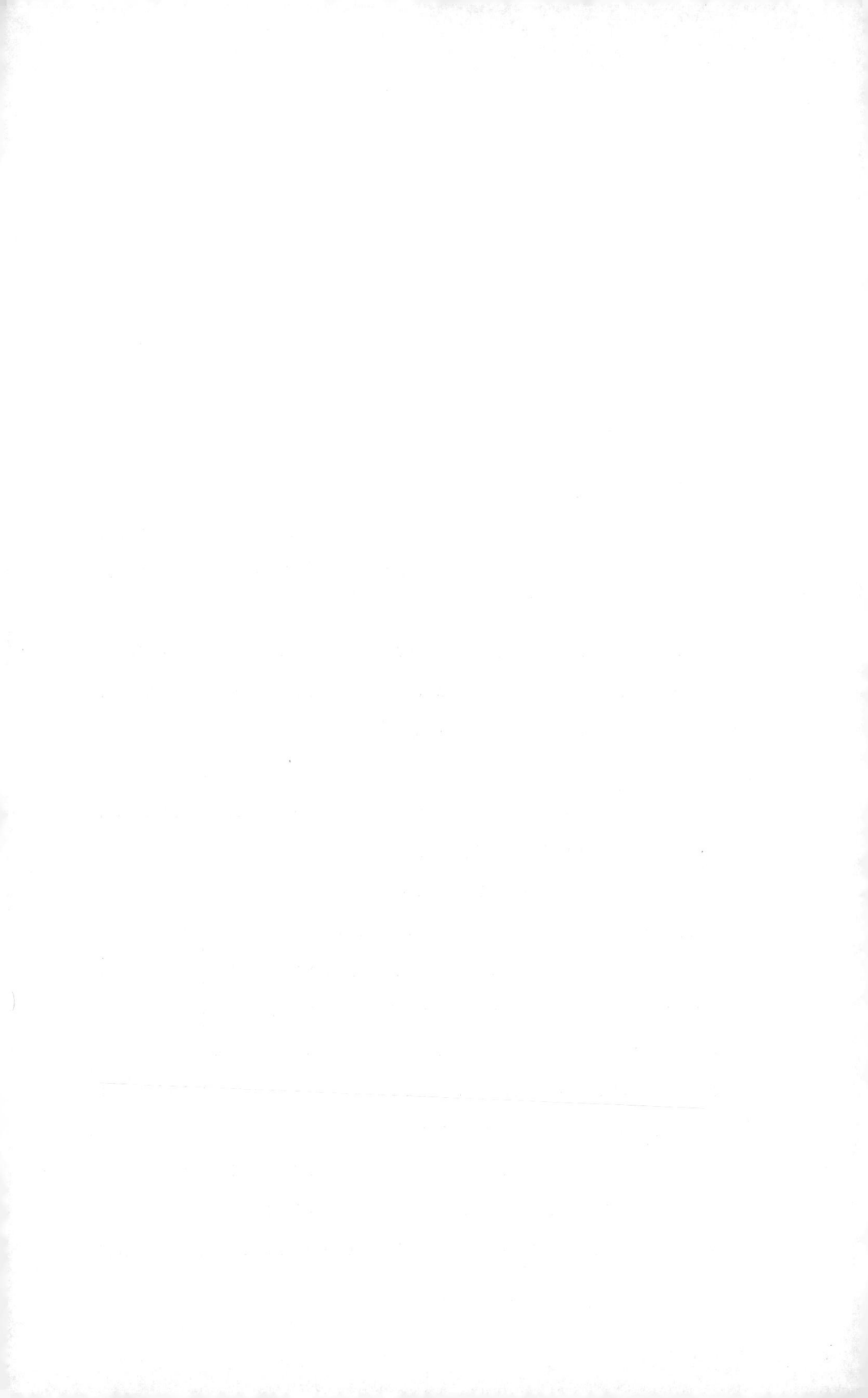

FOREWORD

First off, this foreword will be longer than typical. It is more like a full-length chapter. But I'm breaking with convention, because I have a lot to say about the special woman who wrote this book.

Additionally, be warned. This book does not sugarcoat reality. If you want the tidy feel-good tale with a pretty bow for perfect presentation, this is not for you. *God Did It* does not present a sugar-sprinkled, candy-coated picture of what happened.

It is honest. It is raw. It is real. It is a story of how God can bring beauty out of something ugly.

So I want to start off with the ugly.

I tried to take the clothes down to the basement where there was a big sink. I let the water run. I had to clean Dianna up. It was hard trying to do it, because she was dead weight. She couldn't stand. I was trying to sit her on the toilet and she had feces smeared everywhere. I had to hold her by the waist with one arm and wash with the other hand.

Her legs trembled and she was unable to stabilize herself. I had to reassure her she was okay. She was embarrassed. She seemed shocked and confused by what happened. It was the first time she fully lost control of her bowels and I could see her trying to process what had occurred.

I didn't know why this happened so suddenly. She had not been able to defecate for a long time. I didn't have any answers. Doctors did not yet know details either. She refused to wear her Depends, thinking it was a one-time incident. She was wrong.

There were more accidents. Dianna's defiance made her fight what was going on until, eventually, she accepted the truth. Adult diapers were necessary. I told her she was still beautiful to me and that God was going to heal her. These are the words I shared as I cleaned her.

The first time Dianna reluctantly acquiesced to wearing Depends, I said to her, "You look so pretty."

"I do?" she said and then smiled the prettiest smile. I can still see it.

Then she said, "You're lying. You're just telling me that because you're my husband."

What she didn't know is that I was being honest. I didn't see a feeble, sick woman. I saw the gorgeous jewel I married.

I never doubted that God would heal Dianna. I just didn't know when or how.

I met my sweet wife of 20 years in 1995. We were both at the McCoy Convention Center in Buffalo, New York. We were attending an Official Day service during the New York Western Second Jurisdiction Church of God In Christ Holy Convocation.

After service was over, a group of my friends and I went out to eat at a local restaurant. I had no idea I would formally meet my future wife that sunny afternoon. She just so happened to be dining at the same location with a group of her friends, too.

While standing in line at Old Country Buffet, waiting to pay and enter, I noticed Dianna waving in my direction. Because she was so beautiful, my mind couldn't process or accept that she was actually waving at me.

I whipped my head around to see who else was near me, but no one else was even looking in her direction. Apparently, she was targeting me. I turned back around and caught her gaze again. She repeated her playful greeting from a distance and smiled the most gorgeous smile I had ever seen.

I was simultaneously overjoyed and terrified. She was way out of my league. Could this angelic being be speaking to me, a mere mortal?

I figured it *had* to be a mistake.

Once inside, I walked past her table, gathered myself and summoned the courage to say hello. Funny thing is, I didn't actually try to get Dianna's number that day. Even though my friends were coaxing me to go over there and talk to the popular girl I loved to hear lead songs in the Jurisdictional choir, I waited. I didn't feel the timing was right. I don't know why, but I sensed we would cross paths again.

About a week later, that inner-knowing proved right. After the Old Country Buffet icebreaker, Dianna and I both attended a District Meeting held at Open Door #5 COGIC. Though my mind should have been on Jesus, it wasn't.

The moment I saw her, I pulled out a pen and jotted my number down. I had already concocted a scheme to approach her that night.

At one point, I decided to take a break from the extended gathering. I got up, walked through a door that led to an area where some of the women were cooking chicken dinners, selling candy and other treats. I wasn't expecting to see Dianna.

But there she was, wearing denim from head to toe. All over again, I was mesmerized by her natural beauty as she stood alone near a wall. This time, nervous and all, I seized the moment. I walked over to her confidently.

"Hi, my name is Kenya Hobbs," I said, trying to speak as articulately as possible. I wanted to impress her. After a few fleeting moments of giving her my best pitch, I handed Dianna my red church invite card where I had written my number on the back. I thought my introduction went well, but she later told me I was weird and robotic. No wonder she was looking back at me like a deer in headlights, never uttering a single word.

Well, after she accepted the card, I took all my weirdness back into the sanctuary to enjoy the rest of the service. I breathed a sigh of relief. My mission was accomplished.

Around five minutes later, as I sat with my left hand stretched out over the back of the wooden church pew, I felt a soft touch and a piece of paper sliding beneath my palm. I unfolded the note that came from the vision that had just walked past me.

It said, "My father would kill me if I called a boy. I can't call boys first. So here's my number. You can use it to call me."

I thought, *wow, that's different*. But I liked it. I respected it.

I was happy about having her number, but I was a bundle of nerves. Truthfully, I was freaking out that the most stunning woman I'd ever laid eyes on gave me her digits.

Was this my life?

I was smitten.

I stared over at her once she was seated—that is, until I felt a pair of mean eyes on me. It was one of her brothers silently threatening me to look away. His eyeballs turned into Uzis and shot me down.

When I got home, I wanted to call her right away. But my anxiousness got the best of me. It took me three whole days to reach out. Then, when I finally did do it, I phoned Dianna a half-hour before I had to be at work at the local Family Dollar discount store. That way, if things didn't go well, I would have a legitimate excuse to bail.

Turns out, we hit it off and we've been learning, and loving each other ever since.

Plainly put, Dianna and I are best friends. I love everything about her. She is a sensitive, free-spirited woman and also the sweetest, most kind-hearted, tender person I know. I like to jokingly say that she is convinced that God created the earth out of gumdrops and lollipops. What I mean by that is, Dianna sees things through a lens of kindness and joy.

She is virtuous, warm and trusting. Happiness is all she wants everybody to experience. Even in bad times, she finds the silver lining. Dianna places the needs of others above her own. She is very nurturing and is the humblest and finest representation of graciousness and compassion that I have ever witnessed.

We get along so well and share everything: our hopes, dreams, disappointments, goals, ups and downs. We laugh until we cry and fall on the floor. We play like schoolchildren and generally have a great time together.

She has a childlike innocence as well as a maturity beyond her years. I genuinely enjoy her company. She tells me often that I am her muse and I let her know that she is my queen.

When Dianna's sickness first got really serious, I missed my friend badly. She no longer had the same energy level. The gleam in her eye, bounce in her step and happy tone in her voice was gone. The person I was used to having lengthy conversations with about everything and nothing was lethargic, and barely awake.

Our talk time was reduced to two or three minute intervals in between naps, because Dianna's body was so riddled with pain. She had become too weak to speak on most days. I availed myself in any way I could. I tried giving her comfort, whatever that looked like.

I can remember rushing home from the office, climbing into bed with my suit still on, and spooning her. Sometimes, I'd stroke her hair, hold her close and let her know it was going to be okay, and that the Lord was going to fix it.

Before He intervened, our Friday date nights were canceled indefinitely. There was no more going out to eat, strolling around the park, or visiting local attractions. There was no more stealing away to invest in each other and recalibrate after a long week of work, ministry obligations, and family commitments. The illness robbed us of that. Even though it was a difficult period, neither of us would trade it. It showed us that we have more than fair-weather love. Our bond will hold up in any kind of weather.

Over the past 20 years of marriage, we have remained committed to our vows: for better or worse, for richer or poorer, in sickness and in health. In sickness, I became Dianna's primary in-home nurse.

Some weeks it felt like a blur of back-and-forth trips to the doctor's office, emergency room, and pharmacy. Through hospitalizations, surgeries, tears, and heartache, we grew closer, and made our own sunshine on those grim days. When things went from bad to worse, it seemed surreal.

How had it all gone so wrong?

When Dianna first began exhibiting odd symptoms in early 2015, honestly, we both shrugged it off. Neither of us believed anything major was wrong. On top of that, it isn't in Dianna's nature to accept ill health. Even when she is under the weather, she won't slow down unless illness knocks her on her back. She also prefers prayer over prescriptions and calls the Chief Physician before phoning our primary care physician.

But when she felt increasingly sluggish and started having digestive issues, she went to the doctor. He recommended dietary changes to deal with the persistent stomach problems. Dianna went vegan—no meat or dairy.

For a while, things improved, somewhat.

But as months went by, problems persisted. She battled constant tiredness and frequent colds, and felt funny. Nevertheless, we blamed viruses. Each time, we figured she must have interacted with people infected with some sort of contagious bug, and subsequently contracted it herself.

But then, in mid-2016, the bruising started. White spots showed up on her skin. These marks began multiplying on her legs and grew more pronounced.

By September, I was really concerned. I knew something was off. Dianna's penny-sized bruises grew nickel-sized. When they enlarged, becoming quarter-sized, they spread to other parts of her body. One day, a huge contusion appeared out of nowhere on her calf about the width of the John F. Kennedy half-dollar. A few more popped up in different spots. Eventually, they were everywhere—even on the soles of her feet and in the palms of her hands.

I was horrified.

She looked like she had been beaten in a dark alleyway and it hurt whenever anyone touched her. I knew we had to get help, which I thought would be much easier than it proved to be.

No one could diagnose Dianna for months.

No one.

Dozens of doctors and specialists were stumped.

Nothing stopped the pain or symptoms—not pills, diet changes, or any other natural remedies. As a husband and protector, I went into fix-it mode, but I couldn't fix it. I shifted into problem-solving gear, but I couldn't solve the problem. We each had to lean on the only One who could fix it and solve it.

As we trusted God, we tried to maintain the flow and rhythm of our household as best as possible. And surprisingly, in spite of all of the pain and discomfort that Dianna was experiencing, she never lost her sense of humor. I don't want you to think we were sad every day.

We weren't.

Though it was an especially tough trial, our extraordinarily powerful God granted us peace that surpassed all understanding (Philippians 4:7). We were heavy-hearted and felt overwhelmed at times, but He was right there. On Dianna's good days, which were few and far between as the illness progressed, we still shared a lot of laughter.

Once the public discovered what was going on—something my intensely private wife never wanted to happen—many wonderful people did all they could to help. They sent prayers, monetary donations, care packages, groceries, you name it.

We will never be able to thank God and others enough for the love and support that poured in. When Dianna's body was limp and her spirit was weighed down, I would read the lovely cards and letters sent to her. They came from all over the world. Upon hearing the loving and uplifting messages, she would lie in bed and smile.

I also appreciated those who checked in on me to see how I was doing. I received thoughtful and heartfelt calls, text messages, and emails from family, friends, and colleagues. Some would offer me encouragement as the caregiver by letting me know it was alright to be frustrated.

Compassionate comforters explained that it was okay for me to get away, take a break and escape so I could replenish. They said recharging my own battery would help me come back restored and refreshed, and able to be a better caretaker.

Whenever I received that kind of advice, I couldn't help thinking, *Dianna doesn't get to take a break from the pain she's experiencing.*

Though I never verbally expressed it, because I knew their heart and intent was pure, I felt like, to leave her would be selfish. While I couldn't heal the pain that she was experiencing, sacrificing my time to be a comfort to her was really no sacrifice at all.

It's true.

I never had a single second of regret, resentment or desire to leave Dianna's side. The only time I wanted to escape was when I was stuck fulfilling obligations that kept me *out* of her presence. There was no place I wanted to be than with her, bathing her, feeding her, clothing her and caring for her in any form.

I was happy being a devoted Ephesians 5:25 spouse and loving her the way Christ loved the church, by giving Himself for it. It never felt like an imposition or burden.

Nursing Dianna back to health was not just my duty as her spouse; it was my privilege as her best friend. I was willing to do it for as long as it took for God to heal her.

God did it on March 26, 2017 and did it in grand fashion. It still boggles my mind.

When we arrived at the church for the "50 Women Praying" healing service, I opened Dianna's door to help her out of the car. I quickly reached out to grab her, as she nearly tumbled out of our black family minivan. My wife was feeble and trembling, but didn't want to alarm those who had not seen her publicly in months.

She insisted that we let her try to walk in—which I knew she was incapable of doing at that time. Everyone knew it. She did, too. The pain was severe and she had no strength in her limbs. I knew the whole experience was demoralizing for her. Having others witness her frailty was a nightmarish reality, which pushed her to suggest attempting the impossible.

"Let me try to walk," she asked several times.

Perhaps it was a mix of the drugs, embarrassment and her natural defiance that led to this absurd request. We now laugh at the idea of Dianna trying to pretend like she was okay despite everyone being gathered for her healing service. We were all there because she *wasn't* okay.

But that's her.

Dianna is a fiercely independent maverick. She believes in breaking boundaries and trusting God for the impossible. She refuses to settle and accept manmade limitations.

She is carefree and strong-willed. But not even her strong will could carry her weight on those weak legs that day. Once inside, she continued protesting and resisting assistance. Again, she said she could walk and nearly took a nasty spill before I caught her.

My mind was racing. My adrenaline was pumping. I did my best to stay focused on the main thing: taking Dianna to the King. I made sure we had the children lined up. They had their instructions for carrying several accessories to comfort Mommy during the service: a step stool for her to rest her feet on and a giant pink pillow.

Rarely could Dianna sit up for long periods of time, so I wanted her to be as comfortable as possible.

Finally, we were all set.

Despite her resistance and insistence on independence, I swooped her up in my arms and proceeded to carry her down the aisle to the front. I felt that nothing—no barrier or impediment of the enemy—was going to stop me from getting Dianna positioned for her healing.

We had come too far. Back in the hotel room, after she had broken down and felt like she couldn't make it, through her tears and mine, I told her, "You are only moments away from your miracle."

I believed that with every part of me.

And so I walked into Covenant of Grace Fellowship International in Niagara Falls, New York, carrying my beautiful bride with all the gentleness that one would carry a package marked *Fragile*. I wanted to ensure that she would make it to her proper place, so God could do what He had promised us He would do, and heal her body.

God did it.

I can't tell it like she can, because I didn't feel what she felt. But after affliction was divinely cast out of her body, I saw my wife up, running around the sanctuary, singing, and praising God. It was almost a dream-like experience. I am usually composed and reserved. Not that night. I lost every bit of composure I had. I sobbed. I danced before the Lord. I stood in awe of God's power. He kept His word. He brought my wife, my best friend, the one I love waking up to every day, back to me.

Seeing her completely healed let me know, if I had any fragments of doubt, that there indeed is a God in Heaven, who looks down upon us. He is intimately aware of our situations and can step in at any moment and change the course of our lives. All we have to be is in the right place and position to receive what He has for us.

As you read Dianna's story, I assure you that each vivid detail of the entire account is true. I witnessed it all and will, for the rest of my days, give thanks unto the Lord for what He, by His grace, has done for our family.

Kenya Hobbs
Dianna's Best Friend

PREFACE

I am currently sitting on the patio of my room at Grotto Bay Beach Resort & Spa in Bermuda. It is a perfect 71-degree morning with an ever-so-gentle breeze rustling through the trees. The birds are chirping, vacationers are walking and enjoying the amenities the resort offers. And I, well, I am writing to you, periodically glancing over at the attention-arresting view, mesmerized by God's creation and handiwork.

It is Monday, February 26, 2018, exactly one month before the one-year anniversary of my miraculous healing from two incurable autoimmune diseases—Rheumatoid Arthritis and Fibromyalgia.

I have no pain. I am strong. I am whole—in every way. And I am in Bermuda, not for vacation purposes, but for ministry. I was invited to share my testimony and the gospel of Jesus Christ for three consecutive days as part of the 2018 Women's Weekend Celebration hosted by First Church of God, Bermuda. It was a life-changing experience where deliverance and breakthrough broke out among the vibrant body of believers led by Bishop Vernon G. Lambe and Lady Ruth Ann Lambe.

At present, I have completed my assignment here and am preparing to fly home soon. Before leaving, however, I dug my toes into the cool sand on the scenic beach a short distance away from my room. With childlike joy and amazement, I splashed my feet in the turquoise water on the sleepy island.

I felt so alive.

I also whispered a word of thanks to God for using me to reach souls this weekend, letting me experience this little piece of heaven, and allowing me to survive the roughest period of my life.

Beautiful things really do come from ugly circumstances. Miracles still do happen. That is exactly what was on my mind as I walked around the resort. I thought about God's sovereignty as I breathed in the fresh air. I meditated on His mercy while marveling over this island of paradise, so far away from my home in America. It seems crazy that, right around a year ago, I was fighting for my life. Now I am fighting back tears as I think of the remarkable way God spared my life.

When I consider that I was confined to my bed of affliction, in total misery, a short while ago, how can I do anything but praise God? How can I not give Him heartfelt thanks all day, every day? I am amazed that God saw fit to cure me. I am overwhelmed at the thought of it. He predestined that I would be right here, on this island in the Atlantic Ocean, off the Carolina coast, in the British colony, to tell the good news of His healing power.

In the words of Mary, the mother of Jesus, in Luke 1:46, "My soul doth magnify the Lord."

During this trip, I have seen the sovereignty of God at work. I cannot count the number of women I met who are battling autoimmune diseases, just as I was not too long ago. Their children are suffering. My heart was moved with compassion as I listened and noticed the tears forming in their eyes. I know those feelings of desperation well. They have been crying, visiting physicians, seeking answers and trusting God for healing.

God sent me for them. The Holy Spirit offered the comfort and assurance they need through the word of God. Sometimes, we need confirmation of what we already know. We need to be reminded that the God of the Bible is still doing what the faithless call impossible.

How wonderful it is for me to know that hearing my testimony gave these beautiful Bermudians hope. This entire weekend rejuvenated their faith and helped them recognize that the same God who healed me is willing and able to do it for them. We rejoiced, danced and shouted for joy together; it was an experience I shall never forget.

I believe God sent me for you, too.

I don't know what's going on in your life as you read this book He told me to write. You may or may not have a physical ailment. But whatever you *are* facing, God has not forgotten you. He has not lost your address or neglected to keep His appointment with you. He did not stand you up. He has not made you false promises. No matter how long it has been, it is not too late for a turnaround.

You might be like the woman with the issue of blood in Luke 8:43-48, who bled for 12 years. You, like her, may have a chronic issue. It doesn't have to be sickness. It could be anything recurring, any bondage you can't seem to get out from under. If you have exhausted all options and don't know what to do, I've got good news: just as Jesus remedied the issue for the woman with the issue of blood, the Lord will do the same for you.

I know negative situations are intimidating. Fear tries to weasel its way in. Worry knocks at the door and it's unnerving. But fear not. God yet has power over disease, death, and the very forces of darkness that seek to destroy you. I'm a living testimony.

WHY I WROTE THIS BOOK

I wrote *God Did It: A True Story of Miraculous Healing* to remind you that all power belongs to our God. He is victorious. He is indomitable and more than able to do all things.

I believe this book is the Lord's tool to transmit truth and encouragement to help those who, like the man in Mark 9:24 are crying out, "I do believe, but help me overcome my unbelief!" *God Did It* will increase your confidence in His miracle-working power.

At the same time, through these pages, you will find comfort and answers to your why questions: why the storm? Why the pain? Why the struggle? Why the suffering? Why the unanswered prayers? Why me? Why has this happened? Where is God? Where are His miracles?

If you have ever asked one or all of those questions, the book you're holding is God's response. It is His way of speaking for Himself. He is telling you, *I am here in the midst of your trial. I am who My word says I am. I can do what My word says I can do.* Whether you know Dianna Hobbs or not, Christ is using the hands of this Jesus-loving girl from Buffalo that has been healed by His stripes, to reveal Himself.

I am merely a conduit, telling you to lift up your head. Your situation may be impossible with man, but not so with God. No matter how out of sorts things are, or how hard a hit your faith has taken, God is able to restore everything. Believe that you will recover all.

I have.

This real-life account, which remains difficult for me to wrap my mind around to this day, is a reminder to you that Psalm 34:19 NIV is not a myth. When the word of God says, "The righteous person may have many troubles, but the Lord delivers him from them all," it is fact.

WHAT YOU CAN EXPECT

With each page you turn, prepare to see your faith level increase. As you believe God for greater, He will manifest Himself in greater ways.

So come. Take my hand. Let me guide you through the incredible twists and turns of my journey. Go with me to the deepest recesses of the valley, then travel up to the apex of the mountain. There, you will see the glory of God on full display.

Through seven chapters, each representing a phase in my evolutionary process, you get to see exactly how I arrived at this place of total freedom and holistic deliverance. You will need to read *God Did It* through completely to gain a clear view of the completed work of Christ as it is revealed in my life.

At the end of each chapter is an intercessory prayer for you, so your faith won't fail you in your time of need. Through these prayers, we will touch and agree, and connect our faith. Expect to see God move.

Whether you are near or far, we are coming together in spirit. Jesus said in Matthew 18:19 NIV, "Again, truly I tell you that if two of you on earth agree about anything they ask for, it will be done for them by my Father in heaven."

Whether you are believing for your children, your spouse, some other relative, an individual you don't know personally, a friend, colleague, a group of people, or for yourself, God is in the midst of us. He hears and He will answer.

INTRODUCTION

One December day, a full nine months after God healed me, I had this troubling dream that I was sick again. One minute, I was walking with my husband Kenya on a sunshiny day, healthy, spry and strong. Then, in a blink, my physical condition began changing. My legs grew weak and heavy. My pace slowed. Shortly thereafter, my breathing was labored. I was wheezing and gasping for air, exactly the way I used to after only a few minutes of activity.

I was suffocating on my feet.

No one around me noticed my regression. Everything moved in slow motion. I could see others smiling and addressing me, but their words were distorted and bounced off my ears like soundwaves on cave walls. Why could they not see I was suffering? How come they didn't know I was being physically accosted by an enemy I thought had been defeated?

Severe Rheumatoid Arthritis and Fibromyalgia, the ugly pair that tag-teamed and mercilessly brutalized me, leaving me fighting for my life, had come back in a night vision. Unlike the most common form of arthritis that comes from wear and tear on the body, as well as age, Rheumatoid Arthritis is different.

Way different.

It was in my blood. All in and through it. It was bad. Nothing could contain it. This pair of evil predators haunted me 24 hours a day, 7 days a week. Rheumatoid Arthritis, an inflammatory disease that causes white blood cells to mistake healthy cells for foreign invaders, like bacteria and viruses, ate me up.

Literally.

It was eroding away my joints, bones, muscles, and damaging major organs. To make matters worse, its partner in crime, Fibromyalgia, walloped me with widespread musculoskeletal pain, fatigue, sleep, memory, and mood issues.

The combination of the individually painful diseases made living unbearable. Add the side effects of approximately 13 different medications and you get the perfect storm of physical, mental and emotional torture.

Until I fell into the rabbit hole of hard-to-diagnose medical cases, I didn't know much about autoimmune diseases. Now I know they are a group of diseases that can impact almost every human organ. They destroy nervous, gastrointestinal, and endocrine systems, skin and other connective tissues, eyes, and blood vessels.

I tested positive for a high level of "The Rheumatoid Factor"—a bad protein in my blood— making my circumstances especially dire, and my deterioration faster. I had an aggressive case. My situation worsened with treatment. At the rate I was going, my Rheumatoid arthritis would result in fatality due to serious medical complications.

I was on the road to becoming a statistic.

According to The Rheumatoid Arthritis Support Network (RASN), over half of Rheumatoid Arthritis patient deaths were the result of heart disease and cardiovascular issues. Along the way, I had so many heart, lung, bowel and blood pressure issues, leading to life-threatening episodes. My case had doctors scrambling and unsure of what to do.

When God set me free, He saved my life.

I am forever grateful.

But that gratefulness turned to fearfulness in my dream last December. In my sleep, I was surrounded by loved ones on an idyllic day. Then, boom! All my healthy, exciting progress was reversing like 32-year-old Charlie, the protagonist from the science fiction short story, *Flowers for Algernon*.

Have you ever read it?

When I read it in grade school, I felt sorry for Charlie. He was a mentally disabled man who was chosen by a team of scientists to undergo an experimental surgery to increase his intelligence level. The procedure seemed promising after it worked on a mouse named Algernon. But, by the time the story ended, the short-lived phenomenal breakthrough was too good to be true.

Algernon died. Charlie's disabilities resurfaced. He completely regressed. The adventure was over. The excitement ended. And I, the young reader, was devastated.

I never forgot that story. I knew it wasn't real, but my emotions were still triggered. Why couldn't Charlie be okay? Why couldn't scientists figure out how to permanently help him? What went wrong?

In my dream, like Charlie, my healing didn't last either. In real life, test results have confirmed the sudden disappearance of any traces of my diseases. During this disturbing dream, though, I wound up in the same miserable predicament. How could this happen?

When I woke up, I stared at the wall for a while. It was early. All was still, except my racing mind. Everyone in the house was sleeping, but I could no longer rest because I was perplexed and vexed. God deals with me in dreams, so I wanted to know its meaning. What message was the Lord conveying? It couldn't be that His power was limited and the miracle He worked was a fluke.

I laid stiff as an arthritic limb, waiting for Him to speak. He did and I now I get it. God was pointing out the ridiculousness of Satan's attempts to toy with my mind about the validity of the miracle He performed for me. You see, whenever my heart beats rapidly, or I feel any sort of ache—whether from stubbing my toe, intensely working out, or experiencing a headache from lack of sleep— the enemy whispers, you are not healed. You are still sick.

Satan loves playing that head game with me. He doesn't want me, or you for that matter, to believe that miracles are legitimate today. He hopes believers will stop believing. He wants us all to become doubters and assume miracle season ended when Jesus ascended back to Heaven to sit at the right hand of the Father.

But through my dream, God reminded me that my previous suffering went well beyond mild discomfort and slight achiness. At my frailest, I could not freely move about. Physical exertion literally left me breathless. I regularly wept and wailed from the severity of my spasms and nerve pain. My blood pressure was so high, doctors feared I would have a stroke, yet they could not regulate it. My digestion was crippled and I was losing ten pounds per week.

Doctors turned me over, threw their hands up, sent me home and told me that no further progress was achievable. Successful pain management was my only hope. Basically, I would be severely disabled forever. In time, the numerous complications I was experiencing in my internal systems would snuff my life out.

But God said *not so*.

He delivered me—suddenly and miraculously.

I am not Charlie.

I am not Algernon.

No matter how brilliant and believable the fictional story written by Daniel Keyes is, my breakthrough was not manufactured by specialists' experimental treatments. It was orchestrated by God Himself. And He doesn't half do anything.

Had I never gone back to the doctor to be re-tested, which I did, the instantaneous restoration of my mobility, cancellation of my pain and regulation of my system's functions, was all the evidence I needed. I knew before specialists' shock and amazement at my condition's reversal, that God did it.

I am not the same and never will be again.

Since the Lord wrought a work in me, I have heard ministers, evangelists, pastors and incredible servants in God's Kingdom say, "Dianna, before hearing your testimony, I was growing discouraged, because I wasn't seeing God perform any miracles."

I always get excited when I hear that. That alone makes what I suffered worth it. God is restoring the faith of His people. He is proving the point that Jesus's miracles did not stop after Calvary. The supernatural did not cease after the apostles of the early church went home to be with the Lord. Miracles continue to happen all over the world: in big cities, remote villages, small towns and in diverse communities. My story is one of millions.

Yet, multitudes of people have not witnessed His wonders. Therefore, Satan has used our lack of experience with the supernatural as leverage against our faith. Not bearing witness to a miracle does not mean miracles don't happen. But if the enemy can get us to stop anticipating the miraculous, he wins. If we feel like we are in a spiritual drought in the Body of Christ, we can easily grow jaded and let doubt grip our hearts.

But don't let Satan plant seeds of skepticism within you and hinder your faith. Whatever your storm, through this book, it is my hope that the Son will shine through the clouds. I earnestly pray that the bright rays of truth will chase away the darkness of unbelief and prove that God works present-day miracles.

All people, of all nations, cultures, ethnicities, creeds and religions must know that Jesus is alive. Though pain and brokenness exist in the world, there is a soother and Savior who is more than able to right what is wrong.

I remember when the raging sea of indisposition threatened to drown me. It came to test my convictions. I'll admit that I was, at times, totally intimidated. With darkness all around me, I couldn't see my way out. I heard the crashing waves. I felt the forceful rush of wind taking my breath away. I rocked back and forth on the violent, turbulent, angry waters that stood taller than me.

How much worse must it have been for Peter on a physical stormy sea? I understand how he could step out of the boat and begin walking on water at the Lord's beckoning, only to sink under the weight of fear. His human frailty got the best of him, just as mine did. He talked himself out of the possibility of what Jesus had already made possible.

When this fretful disciple lost his faith-footing, in Matthew 14:31, Jesus reached out to help him, so he wouldn't drown.

He did the same thing for me. This book is His way of doing it for you. He won't let doubt sink you. He's giving you a big boost of faith and saying, *hang on. I am yet on the throne. I am still working.*

Prior to my healing, in the midst of the torrent, I got pretty shaken up and banged up, but I held fast to God's unchanging hand. He didn't let me go down. In fact, He commanded me to walk on water, despite what it looked like.

The Lord is still in search of water-walking faith. When He finds it, He is able to perform miracles. Satan is aware of that, which is why he fights our faith so hard. He knows that as long as we view Jesus as a historical figure that once transformed lives in ancient times, but doesn't do that today, we won't witness His power.

So put your faith to work. If you say you believe, put some feet on your faith. Walk by faith and not by sight. When it storms, walk on by faith. When it gets rough, walk on by faith. When the scary waves roar and crash against your face, walk on by faith.

High tide is high time to expect a miracle. When the storm gets most violent, our faith ought to be more aggressive than the storm. Jesus, who calmed the seas, is with you. Jesus, who robbed the grave, is active. Jesus, who healed the infirmed, is in you.

He is getting your attention.

He is shaking you and saying, *in the modern-day church, I am healing. I am saving. I am destroying yokes. I am transforming. I am speaking through this book you're holding.*

You did not stumble across *God Did It* by happenstance. Whatever the circumstances are that contributed to you getting your hands on my true story, they were divinely set up. It is the will of our sovereign Lord for you to read every word here. Whether or not we ever connect in person, we were meant to cross paths through this book.

You, my friend, like me, have traversed rocky terrain. Our stories may not be the same, but you have survived treacherous valleys. You have scaled intimidatingly high mountains and made it through difficulties of your own. The Lord allowed you to make it to the other side for a reason.

He sustained you and brought you over in one piece because there is more for you to do. You have a testimony that will set captives free. Don't faint. Don't be weary in well-doing. Reaping time is coming as Galatians 6:9 promises.

There are greater works you have been anointed and appointed to do in your life.

In order to reach the milestones and prosper in the things God has called you to, you have to expel doubt and fear. You must believe that anything is possible with God; it is necessary for you to reawaken the faith that is in hibernation like a bear during its months-long winter sleep.

That is the purpose of *God Did It*… to wake up the slumbering giant within you: your faith. Use it as a tool to fuel your belief and the belief of loved ones. My story, though it is not written in chronological order, is divinely ordered.

The narrative does not unfold in a straight line.

It does not follow a set timeline.

It bobs and weaves.

It goes forward then backward.

It is a collection of recollections from my stint with illness, as well as other fierce battles I have fought and won by the grace of God. These pages intertwine various scenarios and life experiences, both good and bad, high and low. It spans many years.

God Did It, in essence, is a beautiful tapestry and an antidote for the doubter. It is a memorial to God's greatness, similar to the memorials erected in the Old Testament. When God performed miracles on behalf of the nation of Israel, He instructed them to set up stone monuments, so they wouldn't forget the monumental things He had done.

God had Israel to mark the territories where He did the impossible. In addition to reminding the Hebrews of God's incredible power, these memorials would also awaken curiosity in future generations about the supernatural events they symbolized.

As the happenings were recounted throughout history, they would become a part of the oral tradition of Israel. Others would come to know God through these stories. This helped carry on the legacy of faith.

In Joshua 4 we see this. Here, the Lord commanded Joshua to pick twelve men from among the people of Israel—one man per tribe. They were told to get stones from the middle of the Jordan River and set them up where they were camping out. In verse 24, God said this was done, "so that all the peoples of the earth may know that the hand of the Lord is mighty, that you may fear the Lord your God forever."

I love that verse so much.

The hand of the Lord is mighty: mighty to deliver; mighty to save; mighty to set free from bondage; mighty to restore what was lost; mighty to resurrect that which was dead; mighty to recover the sight of the blind.

He is mighty to heal Dianna Hobbs of two incurable autoimmune diseases.

He is mighty to lift *you* out of whatever your pit is.

The God we serve is more than able. His mighty hand will deliver.

Whatever you're faced with, whether it be physical, emotional, spiritual, mental, financial, or relational, let the miracle God worked for me encourage you. Though I may not have a heap of rocks to serve as a reminder, I have pages of recorded history to memorialize the awesome deeds of the Rock of my salvation.

1 Peter 2:4 calls Jesus the "living stone," the one who was rejected by men, but is yet the foundation of our faith.

Psalm 62:6 NIV says of the Lord, "Truly he is my rock and my salvation; he is my fortress, I will not be shaken."

The Lord, my Rock, is my healer—and yours.

Are you ready to take this journey and be positioned to receive what God wants to do in your life?

Yes?

Then, what are you waiting for?

Read on.

PHASE ONE

COVERING UP

Concealing what is wrong never makes it go away.

His voice was filled with laughter as he shouted out, *"Moringa!"*

I looked up to see to whom the jolly-sounding, deep voice belonged. I was about to hop into my waiting shuttle, head to the airport, and return home.

"Evangelist Hobbs!" called out the robust gentleman with a kind smile. "We enjoyed you this weekend."

He told me he had been in the service and heard me share my story about the Moringa oleifera plant, which has incredible health benefits and is highly nutritious. While ministering, I shared with the congregation something wow-worthy God did. When my illness got really bad, I could not eat and was dropping about ten pounds per week. Doctors were frightened by the alarmingly rapid weight loss.

When I tried to swallow, it felt as if someone was stabbing me in my throat. It was too painful to eat. Kenya, who did everything he could to get some nourishment into me, would faithfully feed me fruit. At my most critical, though, I could only nibble. It took 15 minutes to get down half of a grape.

If you have ever gotten a fish bone stuck in your throat and swallowed, that needle-prick sensation is a perfect example of what swallowing food of any kind felt like – only worse. Not eating meant I was wasting away quickly. No one knew what to do about it. I didn't want the severity of my situation broadcasted.

I was covering it up.

My family members and friends would check up on me, trying to make sure I was eating. Most days I wasn't. My body was giving up. The possibility of death hung over me like heavy smog.

One day, a good friend of mine, Rhonda Smith from Detroit, Michigan, called me up. I discovered her in 2011 through a writing project. Of twenty-four writers, we were the only two African-American women selected to submit short stories about motherhood for a Christian devotional geared toward new moms.

I felt led to reach out to Rhonda. I invited her to write for my Christian online magazine, Empowering Everyday Women (EEW) and she obliged, becoming a parenting columnist. Her columns were always biblically-sound, helpful and they blessed our audience tremendously.

We have been friends, prayer and Bible study partners, and tightknit sisters in Christ since that time. There have been times when we've talked on the phone for hours. We have cried, prayed, praised and had straight-up church. She is a God-send.

Well, when I was afflicted, Rhonda, who flew in from The Motor City to be one of the intercessors at my "50 Women Praying" service, told me she had been petitioning God to reveal a solution to end my suffering. That's when she had a dream about sprinkling something called *Moringa* over my food.

Rhonda, who is very well-versed in natural medicine and has been compiling holistic remedies for over 20 years, had never even *heard* of this plant. Neither had I, nor any of the specialists treating me.

But God knows all things.

He especially knew that my tendency to cover up issues and hide out when something is wrong, wasn't helpful in this situation. I needed nutrition. It was critical that I eat. Being secretive about my challenges wasn't going to make them disappear.

And it certainly wasn't going to *solve* the problem.

Since I was so tight-lipped about just how bad it was, the Lord stepped in and sent Rhonda out after me.

HERE'S WHAT'S SO GREAT ABOUT MORINGA

It is one of the most nutrient-dense plants in the world. It is an excellent anti-inflammatory food. It has all kinds of good stuff in it. It contains high levels of calcium, iron, protein, antioxidants, vitamins and amino acids.

In impoverished nations, Moringa, where it is available, keeps families with a shortage of nutritional foods at their disposal, healthy and thriving.

After Rhonda obediently passed along this information, Kenya ordered some Moringa online. He then began putting a teaspoonful in applesauce and feeding it to me daily. The Lord knew I couldn't consume food. I wasn't able to get proper nutrition if I wasn't eating a balanced diet. So He invaded Rhonda's dreams so she could pass along this helpful tip.

God truly is mindful of us. He hooks us up with the right people who can be a blessing. He will stop at nothing to bless and favor those He loves. This should encourage you right where you are. Even though He might not bring you out right away, He'll favor you in the valley. He'll whisper secrets in your ear and reveal mysteries to help you on your journey. You are always in good hands with God. He is a protective, loving, detail-oriented, all-wise Savior.

As I often say, *who wouldn't serve a God like mine?*

I know He didn't heal me right away, but He preserved me until the day came for me to be loosed from the bondage of affliction. Of course, we all would prefer to be delivered instantaneously, but we don't get what we want all the time. God doesn't always bring us out quickly. In some seasons, He shows mercy by shielding and caring for us in life-threatening circumstances; God is not just a healer, but also a keeper.

If you don't like what's going on in your world and you want to see change, it's on the way. It will happen. In the meantime, be thankful for God's favor, even in unfavorable moments. He may not pull you out of the lion's den, but He will shut the mouth of the lion (Daniel 6). He may allow the heat to be cranked up in the fiery furnace, but He will keep the fire from consuming you (Daniel 3).

There will be days when you'll have to go through the valley of the shadow of death, but you don't have to fear, because God is with you (Psalm 23:4).

God was with me in my valley, my furnace, my lion's den. To reveal that He was there, He sent Rhonda with a plan to keep me alive until He completed the work. All this happened before I ever met my dear sister face-to-face.

THE DAY WE FIRST MET

I'll never forget the day we finally saw each other in the flesh for the first time. It was Saturday, March 25, 2017 in Niagara Falls, New York, one day before my healing took place. I was staying at the Sheraton Hotel downtown, which was closest to the church. Kenya had booked a room for the weekend. That way, I could get settled in before the day of the healing service and wouldn't have to travel far. In preparation to write this book, Rhonda so graciously let me see her journal pages where she recorded everything about the encounter. I was pleased that she had kept a written record, as I was heavily medicated, weak and in a lot of pain.

When she came into my hotel room, another dear friend, Cassandra Elliott, was there. I'll tell you more about her later. But Cassandra was praying and reading scriptures over me when I saw Rhonda walk into the room with Kenya. I cried. I wanted to sit up, but could not. I tried to communicate, but my voice gave out. I drifted in and out of consciousness, often stirred awake by pain.

That is not the way I wanted our initial in-person meeting to go. I always thought we would hang out, talk for hours, eat, laugh and go site-seeing. Lord knows, if I could have hidden away until things resolved, I would have. I wanted to keep my issues covered up, but my case was much too dire for that. It was an emergency. My pride was screaming, *hide!*

And for a time, hide I did.

I DIDN'T WANT THE CHILDREN TO KNOW

In the beginning, before I was severe, I didn't want our children to know anything was different. Besides, I didn't even know what was wrong with me yet. Nevertheless, my attempts to mask what I was going through were ineffective. I thought I was hiding my struggles. But, like the fig leaves of pretense Adam and Eve used to hide their nakedness in Genesis 3:7, my concealment efforts could not cover up the changes in me.

The same God whose voice went walking through the Garden of Eden in the cool of the day in Genesis 3:8, walked through *our* house. He, Himself, alerted the Hobbs children that something had changed about their mother. One afternoon, our son Kedar, who was 12 at the time, knocked on the door of our master bedroom where I was.

"Come in," I said.

He entered bawling. I mean, he was in *serious* distress.

It wasn't the type of cry where a few tears escaped his eyes, and glistened, as they cascaded down his cheeks. Nor was it anything remotely like those hard-to-believe dramatic movie scenes where an actor, who is having trouble conveying real emotion, squeezes out a single teardrop. His eyes were bloodshot. His face was wet, as if he had gone deep diving in a stormy sea of sorrow. Kedar's chest heaved. He struggled to catch his breath, having barely escaped drowning in grief.

"What's the matter?" I asked, eager to know what had him so disturbed.

"I had a dream you were sick. You had cancer and you died," he boohooed.

God infiltrated his dreams just as He did Rhonda's. As you'll see, the Lord did this in other instances, too.

"Aww, baby, I'm okay," I instinctively assured him in a soothing tone, which belied the internal shock I felt at hearing such a statement. I was only in the beginning stages of being very ill, so I wasn't yet aware of how sick I was.

Still, seeing Kedar, with his typically tough exterior, crumble into a mess of tears, was jolting to say the least. I couldn't deny that something bad was happening. Physically, I was aching. On top of that, I had personally had upsetting dreams months prior to any symptoms showing up.

In my dreams I kept seeing myself walking through hospital halls, frail, pushing an IV pole in a gown. It was bizarre. I didn't fully know what these recurring dreams meant, but I did have a strong inkling that God was warning me and preparing me to go through something.

WHAT DID IT ALL MEAN?

One day, prior to Kedar's outburst, I called my dad, whose name is Joseph, and told him my dream. As far back as I can remember, he, like the biblical Joseph, had the gift of interpreting dreams. Dad had previously told me, "God is going to allow you to go through an attack, but you'll come out of it alright."

An attack? What kind of an attack? Why wasn't God being more specific?

The answer would soon come.

When Kedar came to me all broken up and divulged the details of what he saw in his sleep, mentally, I went back to my own dreams, and my father's interpretation. Throughout my ordeal, the supernatural was constantly at work. God communicated with me directly and through other people. He didn't go silent. He just wasn't saying what I wanted to hear at the time.

I wanted Him to say, "Rise up. Take up your bed and walk," like Jesus said so many times in the Bible before the sick were instantly made well.

There were no such words for me—yet. It was all bad news. My mind went into crisis mode. My thoughts could be perfectly summarized in one line from the movie Apollo 13: "Houston, we have a problem."

"Can I hug you?" Kedar asked.

"Of course," I said, holding his convulsing body tightly as he sobbed into my chest.

"I don't want you to die mommy," he wept some more. "You've got to call the doctor and get checked out."

Kedar's impromptu, emotion-filled visit sent red flags waving. But I couldn't focus on me right then. My motherly instinct kicked in. I needed to comfort him. I reassured Kedar that all was well with me. I plastered on a fake smile, hoping to allay his worries and assuage his fears with a happy outer façade.

"I promise I'll call the doctor," I said. "You'll see. I'm perfectly fine."

I would have to eat those words. I would be forced to swallow them whole, right along with multiple bitter prescription pills, and my pride.

Gulp.

I was *not* fine. Not in the least. My husband Kenya knew it, too. Prior to Kedar's meltdown, hubby had insisted that I be seen by our primary care physician. I wasn't interested, but really did need to go. Once again, God intervened. This time, He used Kedar to get me to budge and seek medical intervention.

I had been neglecting troubling signs, praying that everything would correct itself. But concealing what is wrong never makes it go away. Whether I wanted to admit it or not, there was an insidious enemy after me. I needed professional help to fight. Sending my crying son to me, imploring me to make a doctor's appointment, was God's way of giving me the wakeup call I needed.

GOD WAS SABOTAGING MY CONCEALMENT EFFORTS

You know, it's funny.

Not ha-ha funny, but peculiar-funny.

Though I did my best to cover up my health concerns, our children knew something was up. In fact, it wasn't until after God delivered me, that Kyla, Kaiah, Kedar and Kaleb revealed how much insight they had all the while. I thought I was masking it. I wasn't. My smile was as effective a cover-up as air freshener sprayed over a rotting carcass. Something stank and everyone could smell it.

God was sabotaging my concealment efforts. He was supernaturally revealing a lot of my ordeal to the Hobbs children without me knowing it. He talked to them on plenty occasions through dreams. I remain grateful that He communicated with them and cared for them on every level when Mommy could not.

It's natural to want to cover up issues and keep others out of our business, and personal affairs. When it comes to the Hobbs children, the mommy in me wants every day to be free of trouble in their lives. If I could absorb every single blow so they wouldn't have to take one, I'd do it in a heartbeat.

But God doesn't do cover-ups.

His best work is accomplished through exhibition. He publicly exposes things. He brings them out in the open and addresses them. Our issues, diseases and sins cannot be corrected unexposed. God had to out me, even though I didn't like it one bit. I should have known better than to try to hide.

Had I learned nothing from a previous God-ordained exposé? The Lord had outed me once before in the not-so-distant past.

A colleague of mine called me up one day and said, "I need a favor." He asked me to be a part of this video he was shooting for a Stellar Award-nominated Christian rapper. After a brief discussion, I told my friend, "Alright, I'll do it for you."

Saying yes so quickly was unusual for me, but it was almost as if the affirmative answer fell out of my mouth. Looking retrospectively, I see the Holy Spirit orchestrated this. God was up to something.

It wasn't until I heard the lyrics to the song I had to lip synch in the video that I realized the subject matter revolved around sexual abuse.

Uh-oh. That was a problem for me.

A lump formed in my throat.

My friend and video producer had no idea I had been molested at age six. I had been covering it up for years. Saying yes to the project meant I'd have to deal with a very sensitive and painful subject matter publicly.

THE DAY MY LIFE CHANGED FOREVER

If you read my previous book, *The New A-list: Abstinence Makes the Heart Grow Fonder*, you know what happened to me in 1982. In case you have never read or heard my story, here it is.

I was walking alone down Leroy Avenue, a street in my hometown of Buffalo, New York, on the east side, without a care in the world. A six-year-old first-grader at the time, I was attacked on my way to School #61, about a block away from home.

Back then, in our close-knit community, it wasn't out of the ordinary for children who lived near the neighborhood elementary school to make the trek without supervision. Unfortunately for me, there was a predator lurking, waiting for the right moment to take full advantage of this well-known fact.

It was a frigid day, but I didn't mind the cold chill in the air, my stinging cheeks, burning nose, throbbing ears and numb lips. I was too delighted by the crunch of the snow beneath my boots to be distracted by the unpleasantly common side effects of Buffalo's bitter winters. I contentedly marched, fascinated by my trail of footprints marking my territory.

The glare of brake lights was a blur on the busy, congested street, where cars moved slowly and carefully along the icy road. While some children and adults walked briskly that morning, as if to escape the biting cold, I took my time.

Moseying along, I dug my stiff fingers into the deep pockets of my red winter coat with missing buttons. It was held closed by strategically placed safety pins. Before the heinous act was carried out by the man I thought I knew, I assumed his warm smile was authentic.

I honestly believed he was trying to be helpful when he first approached me to adjust my coat. I felt a little embarrassed and self-conscious, not wanting him to see the glimmer of silver pins where buttons should have been.

But his insistence on bundling me up better, combined with my youthful innocence, led me to believe his claim that he was simply concerned about me not catching cold. He told me my coat wasn't properly closed and he didn't want me to get sick, when, in reality, the sickness from which I needed protecting was his own.

Disguised as a friendly neighbor, this wolf in sheep's clothing was a pedophile with no business being anywhere near children. What he did to me on the grounds of Blessed Trinity Roman Catholic Church is forever etched in my memory.

Of all places, near a house of worship, a site representing healing, comfort and joy, a perverse criminal introduced brokenness into my life.

Imagine my confusion when his hands moved from forcing my coat *closed* to prying my most private place *open*.

How did he get his hands in my panties? I wondered silently.

I HAD BEEN HOOD-WINKED

In my favorite red hooded coat, like Little Red Riding Hood, I had been hood-winked and beguiled by a big bad wolf seeking to devour me.

My, what a big smile he had: the better to lure me with. My, what an authoritative voice he had: the better to coax me with. My, what big hands he had: the better to violate me with.

His unsavory appetite for perversion damaged me.

Suddenly, I was frozen, not from winter's frost, but from a mixture of shock and bafflement. I did not move a muscle. I wanted to, but couldn't. I didn't know how to feel. I was six, after all. I was far too young to fully process such complicated emotions, sensations and contradictions. Even women of mature age have trouble dealing with such trauma.

I heard him breathing, inhaling and exhaling heavily in my right ear, fondling me, doing things to me no child should ever have to endure. His hot, lustful breaths rhythmically blew against my neck that day, as my breath remained trapped inside my tense, immobile body.

How had he managed to privately violate me, publicly, in broad daylight? How could he remain hidden from the seeing eyes of passersby?

Time stood still. I was still. But my heartrate refused to slow. Fear and blood pumped through my veins as I, suddenly a mummified corpse, endured this disgusting assault. My heart raced and broke at the same time. For what felt like an eternity, albeit a brief period, he had his way with me.

I WAS DESTROYED BY THE ENCOUNTER

After running to school that fateful morning, I physically escaped his grip. Psychologically, however, I was caught, trapped and stuck in time. I could not bolt fast enough to tear away from his firm hold on my heart and mind. My spirit was broken. I was destroyed by it.

Absolutely destroyed.

In Genesis 39, like Joseph fled to escape Potiphar's wife's unwanted advancements, I, too, fled. Sadly, unlike Joseph, I could not avoid the attack. Joseph only left behind a cloak, which the adulterous woman was left holding in her hand as he made a break for it.

I kept my coat, but left behind something much greater: my innocence, sense of value, zeal for life and courage to face the world.

All of them were gone.

Nothing was ever the same. Years following the incident, that act replayed in my mind, repeatedly forcing me into a black dungeon of pain and fear.

It choked out my productivity and creativity. Day in and day out, I sensed the presence of the man who violated me. Long after it was over, he continued having his way with my thoughts. I was controlled by the recollection of my molester giving me a handful of shiny coins once he'd finished his dastardly deed. Quarters, dimes, nickels, pennies—too many to hold—were placed in my palm.

All that change could not change or undo what he'd done.

It was his pathetic attempt to simultaneously erase his guilt and buy my silence. The money made me feel like an accomplice. No way would I acquiesce to that.

Though but a child, I knew better than to betray myself as Judas Iscariot did Jesus in exchange for 30 pieces of silver.

I fought the best way I knew how.

I tossed the hush money he had offered into the snow.

I stomped it with both feet, feeling angry, belittled and diminished. I then ran to school.

Soon after, anger and indignation gave way to regret and disappointment, not in my attacker, but in myself for letting him do it.

That's what I told myself.

I *let* him do it.

Like so many other survivors of sexual assault, I blamed myself. I faultily thought, *if I had only screamed, fought back, or said something, it might have been different.* Unsure of how to handle what transpired, I buried the incident.

THE PAIN WAS OVERWHELMING

I covered it up. I didn't want to talk about it. I had no desire to deal with the trauma. I wanted to leave the ugliness in the past and forget, forever.

But I could not.

The little girl in the red coat, the six year old that had been sullied and tarnished, never got justice. The man who attacked me walked away. That crime was never reported. I was too afraid and ashamed to tell.

It wasn't until adulthood that I unburdened myself, broke my silence and revealed the dark secret to my mother. It took many more years and the help of God before I was strong and courageous enough to use my voice for every little girl in a red coat who has ever been victimized by a sexual predator, and silenced by fear.

Now that you know my story, as you can imagine, every time I listened to the in-your-face words about sexual assault that I had to learn for the video shoot, they pried open my wounds.

I bawled.

With red swollen eyes, for weeks, I struggled to learn the lyrical content. I could hardly focus on the words, because the pain was overwhelming. That whole process felt like being stuck in a mandatory class I despised, but needed in order to graduate.

"Who do you think you are/To take what wasn't yours," said the words. "The innocence I once adored/Was stripped away behind closed doors."

I turned the song off multiple times. I had to pause, breathe and distance myself from it. But I couldn't get away. Memorizing the lines was only possible for me through visualization of the incident—*my* incident. Someone else may have been able to rehearse the words and mentally store them with no emotional attachment, but not me. I had to go there.

All the way there.

It was overwhelming and difficult.

Revisiting the place, with all the graphicness of the assault, in order to master the recital of each word and phrase, hurt me and helped me at the same time.

Before then, I had been terrified to face the reality of what happened. I had exhausted years, blocking it out. After physically running away in 1982, I never stopped running. Not dealing with it was my way of dealing with it. But again, concealing something never makes it go away. Denying what occurred didn't lessen its impact.

TOO AFRAID TO FACE MY FEAR

Pain tied to sexual abuse is messy. It refuses to be put into a neat little box labeled *Do Not Disturb* in permanent marker, and ignored. It's permanent mark on the psyche demands attention.

Whether it is sexual abuse or something else traumatic, no matter how hard you try to push the memory away, until you truly deal with it, it will resurface in some form of dysfunction.

The unresolved issue will mess up your mind, relationships, productivity and ability to flourish.

I had a fear of facing my fear that just resulted in more fear. See the cycle? God knew I had to *go back* to take my *power back*.

Once I was on the set of the video shoot and had the words down pat, I threw myself into playing the role. It was even more daunting of a challenge than I expected. On day one, I was a blubbering mess. My assistant, Geneva, hugged me as I sobbed.

I was embarrassed. I like to keep myself pulled together. Yet, I couldn't.

It was a process, but with time, counseling, lots of prayer and working through it, thanks be to God, I stopped covering it up. I submitted it to the Lord and He has used my experience to minister to the needs of thousands of women. Exposing it, for me and other survivors, is one of the biggest steps taken on the long journey to wholeness.

I AIN'T TOO PROUD TO BEG

I have found throughout my life that, whatever has broken me, God finds a way to reveal it, so He can heal it. The truth is, I would rather God keep certain things between us.

I like my anonymity.

I would love it if I could get free and keep the ugly, shameful details to myself. But as the saying goes, "The squeaky wheel gets the oil." If you need something, make some noise about it.

Imagine if the lame beggar would have never voiced his needs outside the gate called Beautiful in Acts 3. Granted, he was begging for money and not healing. But the fact that he exposed a need, instead of trying to cover up his issues, put him in the right position to be miraculously made whole.

Peter and John could have never introduced him to the healing power of the Savior provided he was too proud to beg. His condition wasn't one that he wanted to be in, but it was what it was.

Sometimes, you have to throw your hands up and say, *it is what it is. I ain't too proud to beg.*

Drop those defenses and pretenses. I had to do it. And each time I have agreed to open up about what was troubling me, it has resulted in a blessing. Not letting pride guide my choices has made it possible for God to use my life to get glory.

The messiest, most unpleasant junk has produced the best outcomes, because He specializes in improving upon worst-case-scenarios.

Yours included.

My molestation and battle with autoimmune diseases produced pain, shame and regret. That is, until I gave it over to the Lord and let Him turn it around. He healed me and gave me "a crown of beauty for ashes, a joyous blessing instead of mourning, festive praise instead of despair" (Isaiah 61:3 NLT).

On the surface, however, it was all ugly. The real treasure, the value, the beauty of it, was hidden until God dug it up.

THE LORD EXCAVATED IT

Excavate is a word most commonly associated with construction and archaeology. Basically, it means to dig, break up, turn over, or move earth with a tool or machine.

Have you ever seen one of those big old trucks used for excavations at construction sites?

I saw one recently when I turned the corner of a popular intersection and noticed a fenced in area with piles of dirt sitting there.

I wondered what happened to the tall building I'd grown accustomed to seeing. I hadn't been in this area in quite a while, so I had no idea the city was doing any work on that block. The corner looked unusual without the slightly rundown brick structure that used to stand there.

While stopped at a red light, I eyed the bright yellow digging machine's dirty rubber tracks and long handle. They were sitting idle. I stared at the spot where the excavator's shovel, with those massive teeth, had made a gigantic hole in the brown soil. All the traces of the old foundation were being removed, so something entirely new and much better could be built on that site.

In my life, God does His excavation projects publicly. In order to unearth my covered-over trauma, He digs through the soil of my pride.

He rips out the weeds of dissimulation so He can build an authentic ministry through a submitted vessel.

By the time He's finished excavating, the gems of humility and faith shine through. Instead of protecting my reputation, I consider *His* reputation.

The only way He can get glory and reveal His awesomeness is if I ain't too proud to beg; if I ain't too proud to ask for help; if I ain't too proud to admit to the saints that I'm sick and I need prayer warriors to join together on my behalf; if I ain't too proud to let Him make a public example of me; if I ain't too proud to cry out like Blind Bartimaeus did in Mark 10:46-52, *Jesus! Son of David! Have mercy on me!*

When I got sick, there were various stages of the cover-up. Initially, I kept everything to myself. But as time and the intensity of my condition increased, slowly but surely, an unveiling happened. I now know that's the way God works. It is not His will that our struggles stay hidden in the dark. After all, darkness is Satan's domain.

Shedding light on what's happening neutralizes the enemy's power.

GOD HAD IT ALL ALONG

Looking back on it now, I wonder, *Dianna, why were you so worried about the kids finding out? Didn't you know God had it all along?*

I remember years ago when Kedar went flying off his bicycle through the air. My knees nearly buckled. He was in the early days of learning to ride. Though his skills were limited, he had the courage of a warrior.

"Don't go so fast," Kenya and I warned repeatedly. "You could hurt yourself."

But he went zooming forward, pedaling as rapidly as his short, stubby legs would let him. Over and over again, he'd take off and I would go running behind him, trying to shield him from harm. One time, the little guy got away from me and ran smack into a railing, ejecting his body from the bike.

He went so high into the air, I knew if he hit the ground, he would be seriously injured. I was literally paralyzed with fear. Only my eyes moved. I felt helpless and nearly certain that this family outing was about to end with a trip to the ER. But Kenya ran toward him, stretched out his arms and caught Kedar.

It was unbelievable. I cannot explain the sense of relief I felt. I was too weak in the knees to move at first. But I was leaping for joy in my heart. Our precious boy had flown through the air like a Hail Mary pass. It seemed almost miraculous that his father was there to catch him. When I close my eyes, it's almost as if I can still see Kenya, such a caring father, standing there with outstretched arms. He did whatever he could to make sure his son didn't fall.

That's the way God is. He takes care of His own.

He protects, defends, cradles, nurtures and also, reveals. If I had been thinking right at the time of my trial, instead of orchestrating a masterful cover-up, I would have, without worry, let the Master cover my children.

I was anxious for nothing, the very thing Philippians 4:6 instructs believers *not* to be. If I had done what the scripture told me to and resorted to "prayer and supplication, with thanksgiving," I could have experienced the "peace of God, which surpasses all understanding," that verse 7 promises.

How many times do you do what I did and worry yourself sick over things you can't control?

You think of all kinds of bad possibilities and work yourself up.

HIDE-AND-SEEK

I seemed to be stuck in a sick, twisted game of Hide-and-seek.

Ready or not, here I come, said affliction in an ominous tone, threatening to jump out and scare the kids.

I was being stalked by new symptoms constantly. Disease was the seeker. I was the hider. I wasn't a very good one, though.

It wasn't until several months after the Lord had expelled disease from my body that I realized how ineffective "Operation Fake Wellness" really was.

Kaiah, our 16-year-old, told me she had a dream about me while I was ailing. It was actually more like a nightmare, because, in it, I called her upstairs and told her, "I want to die. I can't do this anymore. It's too hard."

In real life, on my worst day, I would *never* reveal such sentiments—not to any of our four babies. I was very measured with my words at all times. I erred on the side of caution when speaking to them. With my husband, it was quite the opposite. I *aired* everything out. I dumped my darkest, most depressing thoughts into the storage bin of his heart. Afterward, Kenya put a lid on whatever I said and stowed it away for safekeeping. He made sure it stayed out of the earshot of the beautiful children we share and love.

But while he and I were busy concealing the truth, God was steadily revealing it in its rawness. In Kaiah's dream, she said she pleaded with me, telling me that she and her siblings needed me. Our youngest girl begged me not to give up on life.

Heavy stuff, right?

Kaiah is our happy-go-lucky teen. She always wears a smile that lights up the room. She scrunches her whole face when she grins and exudes joy. If you ask me, she and all the Hobbs children are way too innocent to be saddled with thoughts of Mommy wanting to check out for good.

But God didn't ask me what I thought, did He? As Isaiah 40:14 NIV says, "Whom did the LORD consult to enlighten him, and who taught him the right way? Who was it that taught him knowledge, or showed him the path of understanding?"

Not me, that's for sure.

The day Kaiah opened up about this dream, I was completely thrown off. My eyes got big. I was surprised and silently thinking, *the Lord unlocked the door to my heart and let you in?*

I only ended up verbally saying, "Really? You had that dream?"

"Yes, I did," she confirmed and added that she had declined to tell me at the time. Even at 16, she wisely understood that, revealing such a thing would have been too hard for me to hear. It would have compounded my misery.

In that way, I'm happy she spared me, though God didn't spare *her*. In His wisdom, He elected not to sugarcoat the situation. Though I thought it best to slap a coat of happy-colored paint over my wall of affliction, our Heavenly Father scraped it off and revealed the bare truth underneath. Instinctively, I protected the children from the harsh reality of the situation. God did the opposite.

One day, while I was still sick, our youngest son, Kaleb, wrote and sang a beautiful song for me as a birthday gift. The lyrics reminded me that, no matter what adversity I was facing, our God is stronger.

Though he didn't like seeing Mommy feeling so bad, the experience was good for him. It forced him to exercise his faith and encourage Himself, and his mom, in the Lord.

Everybody was growing spiritually.

God knew the trial I was so afraid to reveal would work for the good of our whole family. So He excavated what I clawed and pawed to bury and protect, with all the fervor of a dog hiding a bone in its owner's backyard. The Lord excavated that private, shallow grave and let the children see the skeletons hidden there. He exposed them to the ugliness of my pain and offered Himself as protection, peace, strength and comfort.

God invited the Hobbs children to play along in a proper version of hide-and-seek—a divine one. They could hide under the shadow of His wings (Psalm 17:8) and seek His face for strength (Psalm 105:4).

I was too busy in cover-it-up mode and fix-it mode when I should have been in trust-Jesus mode. I needed to switch modes.

Children are very perceptive anyway. They know things about our patterns, and even if they can't fully put a finger on what's going on, they can sense when something's up.

What was I thinking? Why did I assume I had to shield them? Why didn't I remember that He was more than able to care for them?

God didn't leave them alone.

After pumping a bitter dose of reality through their veins, He became to them the embodiment of Psalm 32:7 NIV, which says, "You are my hiding place; you will protect me from trouble and surround me with songs of deliverance."

Through Mommy's distress, they learned more about who God is. They got a deeper revelation of His character, His ways and His power to uphold us through whatever.

Good thing they did, because life isn't pretty. It's a rollercoaster ride. There are some very high highs; just as well, there are some extremely steep drops into the lowest of the low valleys. But as Psalm 139:10 KJV says, "Even there shall thy hand lead me, and thy right hand shall hold me."

For all God did reveal to Kaiah in that dream about me wanting to end it, she didn't fully connect the dots at the time. She didn't know the dream she had was totally on point.

Nevertheless, after she awakened, troubled in her spirit, our teen said she prayed earnestly for me that day. Unbeknownst to her and me, God was cultivating the prayer warrior in her. He was training Kaiah to cast her burdens upon Him.

He was giving her the kind of experience that will prepare her for the real world, which, from time-to-time, delivers forceful blows.

God, being the loving Father He is and a consummate teacher, grabbed her by the hand and walked her to His throne of grace, so she could summon help for her despairing mother.

I'm thankful Kaiah interceded.

Prayer saved my life. It helped me avoid being permanently sucked into a vortex of despair, depression and disillusionment.

GOD IS CONCERNED ABOUT YOU

What a caring and loving God we serve. He doesn't just care for me. He is concerned about everything that concerns you as well.

And while you may not be able to tell everyone what is happening, talk to the Lord and those you know you can trust.

You don't have to endure that dark place by yourself. Let somebody in. Don't hide. Don't cover it up. Don't be too proud to beg.

You have needs: a shoulder; some encouragement; lots of compassion; plenty of empathy; someone to confide in.

Most of all, you need someone to intercede for you.

Allow me.

A prayer for you: *God, there is nothing hidden from Your sight. You know their internal struggles, their private pain, their deepest secrets, darkest memories, most devastating traumas, and fiercest battles.*

Please help them to always run to You, lay their issues bare, drop their burdens at Your feet, and consult You first. In Your arms there is safety, strength, shelter and security.

Your word says in Proverbs 18:10 NASB, "The name of the LORD is a strong tower; the righteous runs into it and is safe."

As they run to You, I ask that You give them wisdom, guidance and discernment. Grant them relief, order their steps and show them who to confide in; show them those who will be an instrument of comfort, help and a source of inspiration.

In Jesus' name, we give You thanks, Amen.

PHASE TWO

OVER IT
Every test isn't over quickly.

How would I know He is a God of the valley if I hadn't spent sufficient time there? How could I know the Lord favors me in the wilderness had I, all the days of my life, only dwelt in the Promised Land? Valley experience is necessary, which is why God doesn't feed into our every whim to be rescued from it.

He is not moved by our feelings of being *over it.*

There were days when I wished He were, though. While I was stuck in the hot furnace of infirmity, I begged, *Oh please, oh please, get me out!*

I GOT LOST IN THE SYSTEM

During my most recent physical struggle, I got lost in the system at first. I learned I had not attained the level of wealth and social status that warranted prioritization in the healthcare hierarchical structure. Though Kenya and I are blessed, and have good health insurance, it wasn't enough to get preferential treatment.

That is reserved for the most accomplished among us.

When doctors thought there was a good possibility that some form of blood-based cancer was to blame for my bruising, swollen lymph nodes, low white blood cell count, and rapid deterioration, I was referred to a hematologist-oncologist. The thinking was, sending me to a physician trained in hematology, the study of the blood, would help get to the bottom of things faster.

It sounded like a decent plan.

There was only one problem: it was very difficult to get an appointment.

The wait time was a lot longer than I thought it would be. When I was told it would be months, not weeks, before I could get in with a hematologist-oncologist, I crumbled. I was over waiting.

Doctors couldn't treat my symptoms without knowing the root cause. And the opioid crackdown, due to the commonality of prescription narcotics abuse, meant no pain management for my chronic pain.

My primary physician looked at me with sad eyes and told me, "I believe you're in pain, but I could lose my license if I prescribe pain meds without a verified cause."

I understood, but that didn't make it any easier to accept. The longer it took to be tested, the more time passed with me hurting around the clock, without any meds to dull the unbearable sensations.

IT SEEMED TOTALLY UNFAIR

How was it possible that chronic pain sufferers like me could be punished for the widespread abuse of legal drugs? It seemed totally unfair. Millions are getting high for recreational purposes.

That makes it tougher for those that *need* pain management solutions to get them, meaning I felt all the excruciating torture with nothing to deaden it.

I was over it, which is a phrase I get from our teenaged daughters, Kyla and Kaiah. They say "I'm over it" when they lose interest in something, which tends to be relatively quickly.

Come to think of it, all four of the Hobbs children have this thing they do; they talk incessantly about how much they love a particular food, then ask us to stock the kitchen with it.

For a few weeks, they happily consume said food. Then, without warning, everyone simultaneously loses interest. They begin requesting that we don't buy that anymore. They're over it.

This cycle has been happening for years. Kenya and I are pretty used to it now. Our troop can be quite finicky and their collective feelings change like most politicians' rhetoric and positions once they get in office. But the Hobbs children aren't the only ones that move on from phases and fads relatively quickly.

We adults also have our "over it" moments.

When I got sick, I know *I* did. I was over it, ready to move on, within the first couple of weeks. All I could think was, *I'll be glad when these crazy symptoms go away so I can get back into the swing of life.*

In my mind, it was going to be a *1-2-3-done* kind of scenario. I would be under the weather for a fleeting moment and then shake the cooties off. I was sure the ordeal would last about as long as a virus: a week. Two at best.

WAY MORE COMPLICATED

Autoimmunity is complex. Way more complicated than I ever knew. On average, autoimmune-related conditions take 4-5 years to diagnose. Sometimes, symptoms seem unrelated.

I was treated for Glaucoma, heartburn, acid reflux, constipation, joint aches, high blood pressure, and a bunch of other things separately. But there was only one underlying cause: inflammation. Every condition was connected, but no one linked them.

For autoimmune disease sufferers, it is common to go years without knowing what is ailing them. In my case, before identifying the problem, doctors suspected Leukemia, then colon cancer, and possibly bone cancer. But each time they thought they had things figured out, test results came back negative.

It was maddening.

I wanted to pull my hair out.

I was racking up thousands of dollars in medical bills for analyses and experiments that gave no conclusive answers. Having weird symptoms was bad enough, but the pain made everything intolerable. My blood pressure was out of control and the headaches were blinding, and nauseating. The churning stomach pain and indescribable never-felt-anything-like-this-before sensations had me at my wit's end.

SO LITTLE IS KNOWN

When I kept coming back to the doctor with new complaints, no one thought of autoimmunity, despite it being the Top 10 killer and the #2 leading cause of chronic pain.

How is it that somewhere around 50 million people in the U.S. have been diagnosed with an autoimmune disease, according to the American Autoimmune Related Diseases Association, Inc. (AARDA), and still so little is known about it?

With those staggering numbers, you would think a truckload of money and research would go toward understanding and curing these more than 100 diseases. But again, it is way more complicated than I knew. Not very much progress has been made over the years.

That's why, in December 2016, when President Barack Obama signed the "21st Century Cures" Act into law, autoimmune disease sufferers rejoiced.

The $6.3 billion healthcare legislation was enacted to speed up the discovery, development and delivery of new treatments and cures for tough-to-diagnose illnesses. Autoimmune diseases definitely fall into that category.

For individuals with critical cases like mine, time is short. They don't have years to wait for medical advancements to produce results. They need help right away. Sad to say, many don't get a diagnosis or treatment before dying. That's something I didn't know before getting sick.

I might have been over it, but God wasn't. He let me stay stuck in that valley for an extended period of time, despite my cries and pleading. It felt unfair to me.

With a snap of a finger all of my suffering could have been over. Why didn't He command my illness to leave immediately? Why didn't God stop it?

With each passing day, I felt more confused. What was this about? Like a three-year-old throwing a tantrum, I crossed my arms, poked out my lips and shouted, *no fair!*

No fair.

Yeah.

That just about sums up life.

MY FIRST MAJOR LESSON ABOUT UNFAIRNESS

In my early teens, I got my first major, real-world lesson about unfairness in the medical system. Back then, I was among the economically disadvantaged. I was at the mercy of a healthcare structure that didn't prioritize or value people like me.

I wasn't actually supposed to know this discouraging tidbit of information. But a trip to the doctor to address my severe skin issues resulted in me getting an eye-opening education.

The existence of an interesting study was unveiled; I found out that some people got treated while others didn't.

Just to give a bit of context, social research studies are common. In these studies, medical teams choose a number of people from a certain group and randomly decide who gets the medicine, and who doesn't.

They monitor the test subjects and compare the results to determine whether the experimental drug is effective or not. Their conclusions are based upon how the recipients of the drug fare in comparison to the non-recipients.

From there, researchers draw conclusions about the effectiveness or ineffectiveness of the treatment.

Well, when I initially got the memo that I could be entered into a study without my knowledge or consent, the blinders of naiveté came off.

Here's the story: I had Eczema. *Really bad* Eczema. The flare-ups were brutal. The itching was intense, like I had been playing in Poison Ivy.

I'd scratch so hard, my nails would break the dry, hardened, inflamed skin.

Behind my knees, on my elbows, in the bend of my arms, on the back of my neck, on the tops of my hands and fingers, the skin was crusted over. It had blackened and would often bleed.

Taking baths worsened the already problematic symptoms. The water would dry out my skin and start the itching attacks all over again.

On top of that, I was severely allergic to dust, tree nuts (walnuts, pecans, almonds), and also, eggs. Coming into contact with any of those allergens triggered reactions.

During Christmastime, when my parents baked Mexican Wedding Cakes with walnuts, I stayed barricaded in my room. If I dared venture into the kitchen, the mere scent wafting through the air would swell my eyes shut.

My throat and tongue would itch. I'd break out in hives, adding to the issues I already had.

Some days, I would lie down and cry, which was a bad idea, too. My salt-containing teardrops did nothing to help the dryness of my skin. That meant more hives. So, even grieving over my sad state of being exacerbated my situation. I couldn't win for losing. It was a vicious cycle I hoped a medical professional could stop.

I was leaping for joy when, finally, my mother said, *Enough. We're going to the doctor.* I was going to get help for my Eczema.

Now, for some people, heading to the doctor may have been their first response. But doctors' visits were luxuries. We didn't have any money to pay for treatment. That's how I ended up in a medical lottery of sorts, a study that was more like a game of chance, where I was to be an unwitting victim.

I WAS INSULTED

When the doctor pulled up my pants legs and saw the scaly patches covering my skin, he was startled.

"Wow," he replied, frowning and reddening. "That really *is* bad."

I was thinking, *I told you so.*

After leaving the room, he returned after approximately twenty minutes with a couple of tubes of prescription ointment samples in his hand.

"I *was* going to enter you into a lottery," he explained, "but your case is so severe, I'm going to go ahead and treat you."

My mother nodded silently. But my inquisitive nature demanded that I press the good Doc for more info.

"Well, what did you mean when you said you were going to enter me into a lottery?" I said, feeling simultaneously confused and interested.

That's when he told me they put some of the low-income patients in the aforementioned special studies, saying it was so they could receive treatments they couldn't typically afford.

His eyes darted back and forth, making contact with mine and mom's in short intervals. He stressed that the lottery was a positive way to assist the disenfranchised.

Basically, it helped those unable to shell out the amount of loot special medical care requires.

As you are well aware, when it comes to getting the best treatment, money talks. If you don't have it, you're on your own.

It's like Denzel Washington's character in the movie *John Q*. He needed to come up with $75,000 to pay for his son's life-saving surgery that was not covered by his HMO. Without cold hard cash, help wasn't available to him. Mr. John Q. Archibald took extreme measures, creating a hostage situation in the movie.

My case, of course, wasn't quite so dramatic. But still, something felt wrong about all this lottery business. The fact that the doctor could have shaken our hands and sent me home without a cure, despite my need for treatment, felt unjust.

Being an adult, with more perspective, I realize the doctor was breaking all kinds of protocols by spilling the beans. But that didn't stop him. He told me they placed the names of patients in envelopes and drew them at random.

Half were treated, while the other half were to be given the equivalent of placebo, an ointment with no medicine, to apply.

This research-based lottery was intended to advance science and result in a greater understanding of how the body reacts.

Though it was the doctor's intention to be kind, he inadvertently insulted me.

Mentally, I had a wall of defensiveness up. I didn't feel like the nice man was so nice any more. My initial elation at the thought of a doctor's visit died with this new revelation.

I was over it.

I was over him.

I was over this lottery.

BEING NEEDY WAS A DISADVANTAGE

The physician had basically informed me that our socioeconomic status, or lack thereof, stripped us of our ability to choose how medical professionals handled us. He confirmed that there were backroom conversations and secret studies that determined whether or not known cures would be given to the poor folks that were ailing.

What if the heart of "Dr. Lottery" had not been pricked by the severity of my case?

I likely would have been sent home with a tube full of Vaseline, wrongly assuming I had been prescribed a helpful topical treatment.

"Thank you very much," my mother said graciously.

I just sat there, a little aggravated, puzzled and somewhat in a daze.

"They can do that?" I asked my mom after the doctor left out. "You mean it's legal for them to enter patients that need help into a lottery and refuse to treat them in the name of research, without their knowledge or consent?"

For me, that was preposterous, unethical, unacceptable and above all things, unfair.

"What if he didn't change his mind about me?" I asked. I was stunned that he could have just sent me packing, itching, with cracked, bloodied skin, and nothing to relieve my pain and suffering. Mom had no answers.

"That's the first time I've ever heard of that," she said, looking somewhat puzzled, too. Though she wasn't angered by it like I was, she did find it curious.

Even though I was grateful to have received aid, my heart went out to all the people, who, like me, were in serious need of a remedy, but wouldn't be getting one.

That lottery, a practice where doctors gambled the health of patients with light-weight pockets in the name of research, inevitably shut out somebody's child, parent, spouse, or friend from the opportunity to have their disease treated or cured.

Being needy was a disadvantage. Finding yourself on the lowest rungs of the socioeconomic ladder meant you got treated differently, and not in a good way.

That's still true today.

While I know lack of money and position don't make anyone's needs any less valid, or diminish the preciousness of their lives, the healthcare system treats them as if it does.

That day, more than twenty years ago, as Mom and I left the hospital with samples of medicinal ointment, I couldn't get that conversation off my mind.

As we made ready to return home with a treatment that went on to benefit my skin and successfully manage my Eczema, I felt disappointed, and a little hurt… but also very blessed.

Deep down, I felt like I had been favored and that God stepped in on my behalf. When I walked into our home hours later, I had lost a bit of my innocence. I was taught what it meant to be poor and powerless.

At the same time, I had discovered a powerful reality: the love God has for me is greater than a system rigged against me and others like me.

He is devoted to my well-being when others don't care about me. There is a wide societal chasm between the haves and have-nots—no matter what our skin color. But God levels the playing field. His favor makes the impossible possible. He makes ways out of no way and opens the doors man closes.

Aren't you glad about that?

GOD VALUED ME

Later, I sat down on the edge of my bed and applied the ointment. As I rubbed it on, I wondered about kids who were afflicted like me—maybe even *worse off*. Who would help them?

I'd left that routine visit less naïve and more wise. I may not have been able to say it the way I can now, but I knew something. I knew that the world devalued lowly people like me, but God valued me.

His great compassion for me, a poor little brown girl, who would have totally slipped through the cracks were it not for Him, moved me. He leveled the playing field for me.

Isn't He awesome?

My natural daddy wasn't rich, but my Heavenly Father is. The Lord can get things done for me that I can't do for myself. He valued me then. He values me now. He values you, too.

So the next time you feel over it *and* overlooked, know that God sees you and cares.

Had I not experienced what felt unjust back then, I wouldn't be able to empathize with the marginalized, oppressed, subjugated and the lowly today. God was developing in me, at an early age, the kind of compassion and empathy that would fuel my ministry.

A contempt for injustice was birthed. It was that very righteous indignation that would, in the future, push me to start a nonprofit, launch helpful initiatives to benefit the hurting, and partner with global charities for the greater good. I would not be who I am today were it not for that.

I see everyone as equally valuable and important.

WHY ISN'T IT OVER YET?

Why are you still going through? Why are you still circling the same mountain all these years later? Why isn't it over yet? Because the work isn't done. But if you hang in there, God will accomplish His will in you.

He has done it in me.

As I was pointing out, as upsetting as it was, I thank God for that lottery experience. Thank Him for your experiences as well. As unpleasant as they may be, He uses rough spaces, injustices and trials to mold us into better people.

He improves our character, develops our compassion and firms up our convictions.

You may be over it in theory, but you won't get over it in reality until you have learned the lesson. God won't actually declare this turmoil over until His work is done in you.

At Calvary, Jesus did not cry out "It is finished!" until after He had been scourged, mocked, brutalized and hung up for our hang-ups. When God declares a thing to be over, He knows the work is done.

When He healed me, I was ready to receive it. I had learned the lessons from the trial. He was able to bring some things full circle in my life following my showdown with illness. I had matured enough to handle them.

Before He was finished His work, I was crying out for my symptoms to get better. I didn't at all get why they were growing worse. But pain, like an adjunct professor, is a part-time teacher. It isn't always there, but when it is, it effectively instills lessons that improve your overall learning and growth.

Being over it is a normal response. But God doesn't just want your station in life or physical condition to be better; He wants your character to be better.

3 John 1:2 NASB says it well: "Beloved, I pray that in all respects you may prosper and be in good health, just as your soul prospers."

In this verse, John is praying for his friend, Gaius. He expresses the hope that, not only would Gaius prosper, advance, be productive and whole physically, but also, that his inner-man would be flourishing at the same rate. In the same way, God is concerned about *us* holistically.

He doesn't want us to have the outer-trappings and trimmings of success, while we are wasting away, morally bankrupt, joyless and defeated inside.

Spiritual maturation is an inside job. When God refines us and builds us up, what He has first done internally, later spills out externally. That internal work, love it or hate it, is done in the valley.

GOD FAVORED ME

One of my many favorite songs by gospel songwriter Bishop Hezekiah Walker is, "God Favored Me."

A portion of one of the verses says, "I know you favored me/ Because my enemies did try but couldn't triumph over me/Yes they did try but couldn't triumph over me."

Those lyrics are rooted in Psalm 41:11 (AKJV), which says, "By this I know that you favor me, because my enemy does not triumph over me."

Friend, this kind of favor cannot be experienced unless Satan comes for you. You don't know this kind of favor unless you have been under attack. You can't rejoice over this kind of favor unless the sniper aimed the rifle, and the bullet penetrated the dust of the ground *next* to your foot, but missed *you*.

You can't celebrate this kind of favor unless you have been through the valley of affliction and emerged with the very life the enemy came to extinguish.

I know I am favored by God, because the enemy of sickness did try, but it couldn't triumph over me.

I can say that now about being tried in the fire of sickness; but when I was over it, while being simultaneously stuck in it, I admittedly didn't feel favored.

I was crying out, "I can't live like this!"

I wept to my husband and vented my frustrations. With no pain medicine, no diagnosis, nothing but symptoms piling up, I had no recourse in the natural. I was out of options.

But God stepped in and favored me in the valley once more, just as He had when I was a teenager who won the medical lottery for my Eczema treatment.

THE KIND STRANGER

I will never be able to thank the kind stranger the Lord used to give me access to the most advanced researchers, surgeons, specialists and state-of-the-art medical facilities: the late Mark Czarnecki.

He was president and chief operating officer at M&T Bank. Sadly, he succumbed to pancreatic cancer in February 2017, just a month prior to my healing service.

When my health took a turn for the worst, Kenya was an executive at the bank and knew Mr. Czarnecki. I, on the other hand, had never seen or met him.

Kenya had not talked to Mr. Czarnecki directly about me, but some of Kenya's co-workers, who had knowledge of the situation, mentioned my ordeal. They told Mr. Czarnecki I couldn't get in for an appointment for quite some time.

Moved with compassion and empathy because of his own health crisis, the big-hearted banker phoned Kenya. He asked if it would be okay for him to make a few phone calls and expedite my process.

"Of course," my grateful husband said.

Kenya spoke to him on Friday. By Monday, I was seen by a hematologist-oncologist at Roswell Park Cancer Institute, where the staff rolled out the red carpet for me. The turnaround time was amazing. How did the timeline change from three months to three days?

In society, they call it privilege. In the Kingdom, we call it favor. God's favor. The kind He gives out in the valley. That's how the timeline changed.

Mr. Czarnecki, who sat on the board, had rang the executive director of Roswell, demanding that I be seen by the best specialist there right away. He told Kenya, "If they don't treat you right, call me and I'll take care of it."

Kenya never had to make that call to Mr. Czarnecki's personal cell phone number that he passed along; I was treated better than I ever had been at a medical facility. I didn't know that kind of roll-out-the-red-carpet treatment existed. Was I Alice in wonderland? What kind of peculiar world was this?

Though I have had pleasant experiences and have been blessed with great doctors, nurses and medical teams throughout my life, this experience was one-of-a-kind. God saw to it that I received the highest quality care.

Though, ideally, I wouldn't have needed *any* medical care, if I had to go through it, this was the best outcome under the circumstances. I was well cared for, immediately seen, and patiently waited on by the facility's staff.

THERE ARE PERKS

When you are a child of the King, there are perks. Divine favor is one of them. It doesn't guarantee that nothing will ever hurt you. It does not ensure that you'll never feel frustrated and over it. God does not promise that you will be exempt from trouble.

He will, however, do certain things on your behalf. You will enjoy plenty of perks, such as the following:

He will make a way in the wilderness and cause streams of favor to flow through your desert places. (Isaiah 43:19)

He will bless you indeed, smile on you, and be gracious to you. (Numbers 6:25)

He will be there perpetually, never leaving you by yourself, and will go before you. (Deuteronomy 31:8)

He will make provision for every need. (Philippians 4:19)

When you are pressed on every side, you won't get crushed. You might get knocked down for a moment, but you won't ever be destroyed. (2 Corinthians 4:8-9)

When you endure great affliction, it makes life tumultuous for sure. Yet, you get to experience God in a new way.

I surely did.

I realized, more than ever, that He is near to us, whatever the issue. He cares for us and steadies our steps on the rockiest terrain.

I really like the way Psalm 18:33 expresses this idea in the Good News Translation. It says, "He makes me sure-footed as a deer; he keeps me safe on the mountains."

No matter how high the mountain, steep the incline, or dangerous the climb, like a female deer that runs freely up mountains without fear of falling, God also establishes *our* steps. They are ordered by Him, as we are anchored in Him. Life is an uphill journey. The sun doesn't shine every day. There will be dark times. We'll feel over it when God is calling us to walk through it. We'll sense the heat sometimes and think we can't endure it. Don't worry. He's with you.

As I have noted, God's favor doesn't stop the flames; it just ensures they won't destroy us. As the fourth man was in the furnace with the three Hebrew boys in Daniel 3:25, Jesus is with *us*. Just as the Lord walked through the valley of the shadow of death with David (Psalm 23:4), He walks through it with us. Favor has its perks in all seasons, good or bad.

I WAS TREATED LIKE A PRINCESS

You're always on God's mind, whatever the situation.

Psalm 8:4 in the Contemporary English Version says, "Then I ask, 'Why do you care about us humans? Why are you concerned for us weaklings?'"

The King James Version, the translation I grew up hearing most often in church, says, "What is man, that thou art mindful of him? and the son of man, that thou visitest him?"

My own version of the question to God sounds like, *Who am I that you're thinking of little old me? How can such a great big God care about all of the affairs of my life?*

I don't know why He has concern or any regard for me, but I know He does, and His thoughts are good. I saw the evidence of this truth throughout my trial, as the perks of favor continued.

Upon my first visit to Roswell, a woman named Jenine was waiting on behalf of Mr. Czarnecki to warmly welcome me, give me gift cards and shower me with attention. I was treated like a princess.

After completing my first appointment, she even mailed me a handwritten *Thinking of You* card.

Teardrops, one after another, plopped onto the paper. In blue ink, among other nice things, Jenine wrote of our first meeting, "You and your husband, arriving that day, for whatever path the Lord has placed you on, will be an inspiration for me moving forward."

She was actually an inspiration to *me*. I still keep the card stored in the bottom drawer of my nightstand. I pulled it out just moments ago and stared at its orange, yellow and purple watercolor flowers painted by Ann Margiotta. The beautiful card reminds me of one of the numerous ways God was thinking of me through the most difficult journey of my existence thus far.

He used strangers to show kindness to me.

Every doctor at Roswell made me feel like I was the only patient in the hospital and made sure my needs were met immediately. One time, when nurses had trouble finding a vein to draw blood and I nearly passed out from pain and weakness, a male nurse, Ken, put me at ease.

He was one of the finest and busiest medical professionals on staff.

No matter what department I was in during my treatment at Roswell, if anyone was having trouble drawing blood, when we put in a call to Ken, he dropped everything to come and do it himself.

When I first met him, I was shivering and unable to sit up straight in my wheelchair. Phlebotomists had unsuccessfully tried to get blood samples for the numerous tests specialists had to run. With collapsed veins, ice cold arms and severe dehydration, it didn't look like this would work out.

But Ken was undaunted.

He grabbed warm blankets and assured me he'd find a cooperative vein. Pointing and looking upward, he said, "Don't be afraid. He's got you. You're going to be okay."

Ken didn't know how much I needed to hear that as I was being wheeled through hospital corridors, poked and prodded, scanned and x-rayed, questioned and examined. The air in Roswell seemed thick and heavy. A weight sat on my chest. My heart was burdened with the realization that I was in real physical trouble. I could barely breathe.

I was panicking.

The negative contingencies and scenarios swirling around in my head were scary, yet served to make the comfort and level of care I received that much more appreciated. That care was just an extension of God's great love and care for me.

Over it and all, I was still thankful.

After suffering through hours of others' unsuccessful attempts at drawing blood that left me with bruised veins, Ken gave it a shot, no pun intended. It took about a half hour, but he took his time, didn't hurt me and found a tiny, barely visible vein.

When we noticed the flow of red into the tube, we both released a sigh of relief. Shortly after, I was whisked away for more testing.

Having scientists and surgeons at the top of their field responding to my every whim was a dream. It made the worst times more bearable. In all my days, I could not remember being fussed over, doted on and gently handled the way I was by the medical team at Roswell.

Because this wealthy, well-connected and respected banker tapped into his network, I didn't have to wait or want for anything. Mr. Czarnecki turned the seeming unfairness of my ordeal from a negative into a positive.

No, it wasn't necessarily fair that I was sick.

But it also wasn't necessarily fair that I was treated like a princess when millions of others in worse predicaments weren't treated at all.

I had won the "lottery" again.

Psalm 5:12 NIV became real, which says, "Surely, LORD, you bless the righteous; you surround them with your favor as with a shield." He implemented a divine campaign just for me. God pulled on man's heartstrings and gave me access to people and resources that were off limits to me.

Honestly, I would not have known how to tap into that level of power. But God, who is all-powerful, all-seeing, all-knowing, all about showering us with His goodness when life is unfair, and always thinking of us, did it for me.

THANKFUL

Some days I felt downtrodden, but I was still thankful. I remain that way.

I'm thankful for Mr. Czarnecki, who played a pivotal role in my process. And since I'll never be able to look him in the eyes and say I am overwhelmed with gratitude, I frequently whisper *thank You* to God for sending him to me.

In fact, I tell the Lord thank You often, for various things: for advocating for me; for causing all things to work together for my good; for sending the gentlest strangers, time and again, to reassure me; for letting me know, when I felt forsaken, that He was always there.

I'm thankful that He showed me that life's seeming unfairness could in no wise outweigh His goodness; for securely holding my fragile heart until the day He healed my fragile body; for teaching me that it is neither money, power, nor access to society's so-called upper crust that guarantees wholeness, happiness and advantages; for letting this trial teach me that it is His unmerited favor and free-flowing grace that preserved my life.

Looking back on it, I never thought I would say it, but I am thankful for that storm.

I was over it early on, but now, having survived it, I wouldn't change a thing. It made my relationship with God more intimate, my bond deeper and my faith steadier.

It reinforced how important I am—that we all are—to God.

He is thinking of me and you all the time.

Being over it, for a time, blinded me to all the ways trials are beneficial teachers. One of the preeminent lessons I learned is, even without money stacks and certain key contacts, my connection to God gets me where I need to be.

God, alone, is enough.

All by Himself.

I see that being looked after by elite doctors and given the most advanced research-based treatments, is not what healed me. No matter how smart various medical professionals were, they could not figure out how to cure me.

For all their helpfulness, they could not do enough to overcome the health battle raging within.

Mr. Czarnecki and all who cared for me were vessels God used to show me His constant, faithful love. They were not the ultimate cure, but rather, their attentive, caring and kindhearted service was a demonstration of God's favor.

All praise and glory belongs to the Lord for the great things *He* has done.

***A prayer for you:** God, in moments when Your servant is feeling over it, tired, weary, worn and unable to continue on, I pray that You will give them strength. Assure them that You have an appointed time for their breakthrough.*

Even when they feel alone, let them know You are there, covering them, carrying them and preserving them until their set time arrives. I come against the victim mindset. I rebuke the stronghold of depression, discouragement and disillusionment.

Though the times and seasons are in Your hands and none of us can predict how long the struggle will last, remind them that there is an expiration date on this trial.

I agree with them now for release and breakthrough. I know You will bring them over every hurdle and cause them to triumph for the glory of Your name.

In Jesus' name, we give You thanks, Amen.

PHASE THREE

ASKING WHY

Sometimes you'll know why. Sometimes you won't.

An ER doctor told me I should consider counseling or treatment for anxiety. "Your blood pressure spike and your heartrate seem to indicate you may be suffering with something emotional or psychological," he said.

On numerous occasions, after months of unsuccessful emergency room visits, physicians and nurse practitioners were grabbing at straws. I had a health conundrum they could not solve.

By degrees, very gradually, the tone of the conversation changed.

One by one, doctors stopped searching for physical causes of my pain, and began propagating the theory that my mind was playing tricks on me.

I could see how we got there. Very intelligent, accomplished, experienced physicians were trying their best to identify the problem, but their best efforts proved inadequate.

What were they to think?

When their research and testing yielded no answers, they wrote me off as emotionally disturbed because they couldn't figure me out. I was told I was likely suffering from "White Coat Syndrome," when a patient's blood pressure rises due to anxiousness about being treated.

"Are you nervous or uncomfortable around doctors?" they'd ask me.

No matter how many times I said, "No, I'm not uncomfortable," they were skeptical. After constantly hearing doubtful doctors' evaluations about my mental and emotional condition potentially fueling my physical manifestations, I felt conflicted. I didn't understand.

HOW DID NERVES CAUSE ALL THIS?

If I wasn't actually sick, then, why was all this happening? How could being a little nervous about going to the doctor cause low white blood cell count, bruising, extreme constipation, joint swelling and erosion, alarming blood pressure spikes that couldn't be regulated with multiple medications, migraine headaches, consistent respiratory issues, chronic pain, insomnia, night sweats, and multiple other problems?

That didn't make any sense to me. How could nerves cause all this?

Deep in my heart, I knew it wasn't a mental malady. But doctors' words are weighty. What they said messed with me a little. I was in a vulnerable place.

I started thinking, *maybe what they're saying about me isn't that farfetched.*

After all, there are real cases where patients' physical problems stem from mental issues.

Then, sometimes, the source of the upheaval is actually *spiritual,* like in the biblical account found in Mark 5:1-20. The Bible says a man lived in the graveyard. He was so out of control, he had been chained up, but even chains on his hands and feet couldn't hold him. No one was strong enough to subdue him. He screamed and cut himself with sharp rocks and was likely written off as mentally insane, even though his condition wasn't a matter of the mind.

IT WAS DEEPER THAN THAT

There was a deeper ordeal—one that it took Jesus to uncover. Demonic oppression was the cause of the man's erratic behavior, and once Christ cast that legion of demons of out him, he was a new man. The next time his countrymen saw him, the word of God says, he was clothed and in his right mind.

His issue, on the surface, seemed mental. But it was spiritual, as was mine. I, of course, wasn't possessed by demons, but I *was* under spiritual attack, despite the doctors' way-off assumptions. The results of that spiritual battle showed up in the form of a physical battle in my life.

Satan wanted to take me out through my illnesses. Had it been up to doctors to cure me, I would have been in trouble. Medicine was not the answer, although God did use conventional methods to relieve some ailments. There was more to my situation than what could be seen. *That's* why it took a prayer service and not a physical procedure to loose me from the bondage of affliction for good.

Back in the earlier days, when I was on the hunt for answers, I thought a practical approach was best, so I was considerably miffed at not being understood by doctors.

Why can't they see? I wondered. *Why won't God reveal it?*

It was bad enough that I hurt the way I did, but when I went to the folks that should have been able to help me, they looked back at me blankly. It was awful.

I went through an extended phase when my very real, but invisible diseases were ripping me to shreds, pulverizing my organs, lashing and thrashing my body. I wish I could adequately explain how terrible it felt to be hurting and not heard; suffering and not seen; crying out for help and not believed. But words escape me. I felt invisible, abandoned and forsaken. But God saw me.

THEY STILL DON'T KNOW

Whenever I'd come back from a hospital visit, all the children would be waiting in the kitchen for Mommy to enter through the side door, the established entryway of the house. They wanted answers.

"What did the doctors say?" they'd ask.

"Do they know what's wrong yet?" they questioned.

My response was the same: "They still don't know."

Our oldest daughter Kyla, whom I call "Ky-bear," helped hold things together around the house as my strength left me. When mobility issues manifested, everyday tasks were difficult to complete. I'd be at the kitchen counter making something to eat, and without warning, like a tree falling in a forest, I'd topple over.

Before slamming into the floor, Kyla would be there to catch me. It was as if a physical hand had chopped me behind the knee. The force of impact caused me to lose my balance. I felt ashamed when that happened, but even more so, I was perplexed. With no diagnosis and with being told that it was all in my head, the situation took its toll on me in more ways than one.

Why couldn't I stand up straight? What was going on with my knees? Why did they buckle and just give out at random times? How come they were swelling? Why were my legs shaking and weak? For what reason could I no longer walk at a normal pace? What was up with me?

Kyla would say, "It's okay," and do whatever she could to help stabilize me. She was and is always attentive, gentle, sweet and responsible. She took Daddy's orders and made sure I ate, even if I didn't want to. She'd make dinner. She and Kaiah kept the house neat and tidy. Like two little women, they marched around, keeping things in order.

All four of our precious ones stepped up in some way. They each jumped on the make-mom-do-right bandwagon. They wanted me drinking water, consuming soup, gulping down healthy smoothies, and getting plenty of rest.

Had I known why I was having these symptoms, though the trouble they caused would have been painful still, I may have coped better. To this day, doctors can't tell me why my immune system turned on me. They still don't know.

In life, we don't always get to know why.

If having answers becomes the prerequisite for placing confidence in God's good plan, well, that's a slippery-slope. That line of thinking trips us up and causes our faith to take a hit, because, plainly put, life just doesn't make sense all the time.

WHY DIDN'T I DIE?

Some years ago, I was on my way to a speaking engagement in Binghamton, New York, and met a fellow traveler. I looked up from reading my Bible and saw a pair of green eyes peering at me over the seat in front of me. The blonde-haired teen, with rosy cheeks, seemed intrigued. She quickly began firing off several general questions.

"What are you reading?" she asked. "The Bible," I replied, which struck up a discussion about faith, Christianity, Jesus and His love. For a while, the conversation remained surface level because she shot off questions in rapid succession, not giving me a whole lot of time to respond. But, after a while, the pace slowed and our chat went deeper.

She spoke of her personal struggles and the difficult challenges she was facing at home. She admitted being a wayward, disrespectful daughter that hurt her parents with her words, and pushed her family members away.

I listened silently. I could tell she needed to unburden herself without judgment. Interestingly, these impromptu exchanges happen a lot when I'm traveling. Random people gravitate toward me. They seem comfortable sharing their life stories. I always view these moments as divine encounters and am humbled that God sees fit to use me in any way at all.

As she talked, she turned red as a rose in full bloom and broke down crying. "I feel like no one loves me and I just want to die," she said between heaving sobs. Since no one was occupying the seat next to me, she slid into the empty space.

"Why do you want to die?" I asked in hushed tones when she came closer. "Don't you know God loves you and cares about you?"

I saw this as the perfect opportunity to witness to her about the work of Jesus Christ on the cross. I told her all about how He died and rose for us because He loves us unconditionally. Despite my efforts to convincingly convey the gospel, she remained unconvinced that the heart of Jesus was big enough to love her. She told me what a terrible person she was and how she felt unlovable.

I asked what she believed she had done that made her unworthy of His undiscriminating love. With that question, we finally got somewhere. I got past the surface and hit the bedrock of her distress. She bared her soul and unlocked a horribly painful memory.

Here's what happened. She and several of her friends were on their way to hang out. They had planned to carpool, but there wasn't enough room for all of them in one car, so they split up. Everyone, except her, piled into the vehicle up ahead. She trailed them, driven by a chaperone.

The driver of the first car lost control and wrecked as she watched the tragedy unfold. There was not a single survivor of the crash.

All of her friends were gone in an instant and her life changed forever.

With that catastrophic visual replaying in her mind constantly, no wonder she was traumatized.

"Why didn't I die?" she wanted to know.

"Why did God let me survive?" she asked.

Her inquest made me swallow hard. This was a tough one. This poor girl cried so hard, it triggered a coughing fit. She gasped for air, gagged, held her head in her hands, and finally collapsed over into my lap. She drew her knees into her chest and wept sorely. I let her get it out. She needed a good old cathartic cry.

"Why didn't I just die with them?" she asked again, riddled with guilt. I learned that deep grief contributed to her suicidal urges, depression and feelings of unworthiness. She had not gone to counseling. She had run away from home to escape the memories, family tensions and overall unhappiness of her life.

Her story grabbed my heart and squeezed. My chest tightened as I prayed and ministered to her. I was trying not to break down. What help would that be? Though I could in no wise explain why the tragedy happened, I *did* tell her who she needed to run to. His name is Jesus.

I believe God dropped this wandering soul into my lap, literally and figuratively, not to help her understand why, which no one will ever know, but so that she could find some semblance of peace. My role was to point her to the pathway to healing. I was meant to use my voice to share the gospel that day. By the time we finished conversing, she looked like a new person. Cheerfulness replaced her gloominess. She gleamed with joy and thanked me for being there for her.

We don't always get to know why. But we can all get to know who—the man that gets us through everything victoriously— if we seek Him.

SHE KNEW I WAS FADING

One night I knew my life was slipping away. It was just a few weeks before my healing service. It could have, well, should have, been the end. I was sliding down the wall in my master bathroom, losing consciousness. My mother was praying over me over the phone, a memory she and I still discuss.

That night, I frantically dialed her number, though I couldn't really talk.

Mom has since told me she knew I was fading.

I pressed my ear against the receiver, listening to her impassioned pleas for Heaven to respond.

History is replete with examples of faith-filled Kingdom warriors that went home to be with the Lord despite praying to stay. Satan wanted me to be one of them.

But my mother and father weren't having it that evening. They rushed over to my house. Daddy, despite being over 80, bolted up the stairs to my bedroom so fast. He had anointing oil and a prayer cloth in his hand, and rebuked the hand of the enemy. It was all-out war.

I don't know when it happened, but the death grip Satan had on me loosened that night. I felt myself coming back.

My heart slowed.

My breathing regulated.

The fog I was in cleared.

The nausea subsided.

My embattled system got a cease-and-desist command from Heaven, and had to obey. I slept like a baby and woke up in the morning with a smile. I thought, *Whew! Thank God that's over.*

But the symptoms weren't alleviated permanently. Days later, I was in the ER, feeling deflated and agitated. I was unable to breathe. They put me on oxygen and administered treatment intravenously. Though I had a sophisticated medical team at Roswell and other specialists in private practices working on my case, too, there were always those late-night emergencies.

I'd wind up at the closest ER, needing a quick solution. Each time, they did all they could to bring my skyrocketing blood pressure down and regulate my heartrate. When my levels normalized and I'd escape the danger zone again, it was only matter of time before the whole process would be repeated.

THE NEXT LEVEL

At the beginning, when emergency rooms first became second homes, I didn't have an outside medical team. I just kept hoping that, with each visit, whatever ER doctor was working at the time, would stumble upon the answer.

Needless to say, this never happened.

That's when I was told I needed to go to a highly specialized hospital. Doctors in the ER were limited in the kinds of tests they could run. If I didn't get myself checked out at a place with more sophisticated technology and testing, I'd keep getting dubious results. I would continue to hear, "The tests were inconclusive. Sorry."

It was time to take things to the next level.

Friend, when trouble goes to the next level in your life—and it will happen—that means it's time to take your faith to the next level, too.

My mind was whirring. My head was spinning. My emotions were raging. My heart was pounding. My spirit was praying. My world was turning upside down. But I did my best to cling to my faith.

WE ALL NEEDED HELP

In the months that followed, Kenya would have to help me shuffle through the hallways of multiple hospitals, imaging centers and laboratories.

Together, we'd pass the rooms of many other afflicted persons. Some were moaning, others were crying, most looked dazed. I didn't know what their problems were, but we were all united by our need for help.

No matter our race, ethnicity, religion, or status, we were sick. We had issues that needed to be resolved.

Spending so much time in and out of medical facilities gave me a clearer perspective. I saw up close how sickness, tragedy and loss unite disparate groups. No one goes through life unscathed.

The tragic trio—hurt, heartache and heartbreak—don't discriminate or pass over anyone. You can't slide by them without being wounded at some point.

That's just the way it is.

As the French aptly say, C'est la vie, meaning, that's life, or such is life.

The French may have coined that phrase, but Jesus already told us, "In this world you will have trouble." He gave that matter-of-fact assurance in John 16:33. That may seem like depressing news. But it's not supposed to be. In the latter part of that verse the son of God says, "But take heart, because I have overcome the world."

When you feel overwhelmed by negative emotions and feelings of uncertainty while on the road to destiny, remind yourself that Christ has overcome all opposition, and you are victorious through Him.

Keep that in mind because, again, you *will* have trouble. That's life. But remembering that you are triumphant already, will influence your response to the negative realities you cannot control.

Let God be your focus-shifter and His word your perspective-shaper. That's how to make it through tough times and come out on the other side of them whole. Intimacy with God, plus understanding and application of His life-giving word, makes the difference.

Without sweet, authentic intimacy and communion with the Father, you may survive physically, but psychologically, you will be damaged. Without Him, you may do the time so-to-speak, but long after the prison cell of trouble and affliction opens, you will remain locked up mentally, and bound by past trauma.

Whether you're experiencing failure in your health, or some other area, let God shape how you see it.

I often tell readers of my blog, view struggles through the lens of God's word.

The *why* of it all, as I've stated, won't always be apparent, and the low points in life are unavoidable. But whatever happens, keep your eyes above and have faith that all things are working together for your good, according to Romans 8:28.

AN IMPORTANT CONVERSATION

These days, when I tell folks how I got over, it's to inspire them to see that, through Christ, they, too, can overcome. Jesus is the focus. That's why my book is not called, *I made it*, but, *God did it*. I don't ever want anyone to think about my story apart from *His* story, for without Him, I would not be here.

But several years ago, I had it backwards. I was wrong. *Wrong about what*, you ask? Well, I didn't understand the purpose behind why I shared my testimony. I had my why wrong. But not anymore.

At that time, I was made aware of my error a few weeks after carrying on a discussion at my parents' kitchen table with my younger sister LaQuinte'. I simply call her Quinny. She was in from Atlanta, where she resides.

After the initial sisterly greetings, our table chatter quickly moved from the shallow pond of small talk into a deep ocean of substantive discourse. We effortlessly swam through various waves of discussion topics, only briefly coming up for air before diving back in.

Somehow, we plunged into the subject of sexual violation and the importance of sharing our stories.

Quinny, also a sexual assault survivor, made the point that opening up about emotional scars that God has healed, directs the attention of the hearer to His power. We each agreed that when others see the hurdles we have overcome, they will be encouraged to believe they can get over theirs. We agreed that there is power in speaking out.

Dad, however, did not fully agree. Consequently, a 30-minute philosophical and theological discussion followed. "It's not your story that makes the difference in people's lives," Dad said.

I jumped in. "Yes, but—" Dad cut me off and added, "It is the *gospel* that makes the difference." I nodded in agreement, eager to expand upon that argument.

"Telling your story is an important part of winning others to Jesus, Dad," I countered.

Quinny and I, like synchronized swimmers, precisely mirrored the other's viewpoint. The two of us were determined to convince Dad to see things *our* way—an impossible feat, mind you. Bishop Brinson is stubborn. Even so, we were on a mission to broaden his perspective.

"It's all about the Lord," Dad said, leaning forward in his chair. "The gospel on its own is enough to draw people to Jesus and change their lives."

I went on, "I get that, Dad. And still, God uses our stories so He can be glorified through them, right?" I anchored this view in Hebrews 12:1 that says "we are surrounded by such a great cloud of witnesses," or, in other words, we have wonderful models of faith in biblical history.

In Hebrews 11, known as the "Faith Hall of Fame," it lists a veritable who's who of believers that famously clung to the promises of God despite adversity like Noah, Abraham, Sarah, Jacob, Joseph, David, Moses and more. In my debate with Dad, I directed him to the testimonies of our biblical heroes.

After about twenty more minutes, finally, we came to a fragile consensus. Personal stories are in order, as long as they point to the most important story of all. I felt satisfied. It was over ... or so I thought.

I HAD MY WHY WRONG

One day, weeks later, while listening to someone talk about Jesus and how westernized evangelicals, or American Christians, focus more on ourselves than we do the redemptive work of Christ, God revealed something to me about myself.

I thought testifying was important—and I was right about that—but I had my *why* wrong. Let me explain. I assumed that liberation came through speaking out, as if there were some intrinsic power in sharing. But that way of thinking overshadowed the work of the cross, which should always be the impetus behind my transparency.

For years, I had focused on how survivors could take their power back by lifting their voices. I shared what I went through, the way I was violated, and how what that predator did to me was unfair.

I talked about my years of sadness, anxiety, fear of intimacy, unforgiveness, bitterness and anger. Those details were in the forefront when Jesus should have been center stage.

Testifying is not to inspire others to speak out and thereby overcome by using their voices; there is no power in our voice alone. There is no power in my testimony unless it focuses on how others can overcome, just the way I did, *through Christ*.

He is the only way.

There is no self-help book, no natural remedy, no practical solution, and no motivational philosophy that can accomplish what He can. Jesus is the way, the truth and the life (John 14:6). The only way to the Father—and to wholeness—is through Him.

Revelation 12:11 NIV says, "They triumphed over him by the blood of the Lamb and by the word of their testimony." If you want to defeat the enemy, the blood of the Lamb is first.

We only have a testimony because Christ, the spotless, perfect Lamb of God, who takes away the sins of the whole world, and conquers our enemies by His sheer power, shed His blood.

The power lies in His blood, which makes the testimony possible. There is no true freedom except through Christ.

Because He took a crown of thorns upon His head; because the nails pierced His hands and a spear went through His sides; because He hung under the beaming sun, miserable from the sweltering heat, unrelenting pain, and debilitating exhaustion; because He longed for the fellowship of His Father, while enduring the shame of the cross; because of Him, I am free.

Jesus is the reason for my liberation. He is the star of my story. There is no reason to tell it if it is not to draw others to Him.

That's why I testify: to witness to others about the power of Christ.

I will never get my why twisted again.

A PAINFUL LOSS

When I was in my early twenties, I was sold out to Jesus, but didn't have a whole lot of life experience. I was preaching the gospel enthusiastically. I taught that Jesus could heal all diseases and hurts, and believed it to my core.

But I was not ready for the kind of hurt I was about to go through.

Kenya and I lost our first child—something that ripped my heart right out of my chest. It all started when, one day, I began spotting. I wasn't in any pain, but I hadn't had my menstrual cycle in months, so why was I bleeding? I called my mother and told her my symptoms. She advised me to call my OBGYN straight away.

When I was given a same-day appointment, I was hoping for the best. Truthfully, I didn't expect anything bad. I was four months pregnant. I was confident that I was out of the danger zone. You know, I'd made it past my first trimester, and since over 80 percent of miscarriages happen within the first three months, I felt safe.

Besides, everyone else told us that, when we entered the second trimester, we were all good.

Overjoyed about our blessing on the way, we purchased things for our new bundle. Loved ones had given us gifts for our firstborn. Family and friends were eagerly counting down the days until the arrival. My small belly had started protruding. I'd already experienced the exciting first tangible signs of life: baby's gentle flutters and kicks.

I was on my way to church when that happened. I jumped, startled at first. Then I giggled. It was the happiest Sunday of my year!

But all that eager anticipation was short-lived. Spontaneously, my bubble of happiness popped. My body couldn't carry the child. That life in me ended. It felt like my life was over.

I had no answers. My obstetrician couldn't explain what happened. This was one of those times I didn't get to know why. Not even my favorite nurse practitioner, Judy, could tell me what went wrong.

"These things just happen," I was informed.

I didn't want to hear that. I wanted someone to tell me they'd made a mistake and our baby was fine. No such news would ever come.

I had not known that depth of sadness prior to losing a baby. That hollowness, the emptiness, the void it left was inexplicable.

A piece of me was missing. Gone forever. Miscarrying leaves a hole in the soul.

My older brother, Dion, didn't know what to say. So he stopped by our tiny apartment and left a gift outside the door. It was a sympathy card and a pack of Oreo cookies, the sweet treat I'd craved throughout my short pregnancy. When Kenya brought the card and cookies to me, I shed so many tears. I appreciated Dion's gesture, but my heart was broken. Kenya's was, too. He cried as hard as I did. We both sat on the floor, bawling.

"My baby, my baby, my baby," I sobbed. "Why did God take my baby?"

Neither the sweetness of Dion's gesture, nor of the snack he purchased for me, could overpower the bitterness of that loss. I fell into a deep depression. I never imagined I would leave the hospital in a haze, engulfed in a fog of devastation.

I refused to eat or drink. I could not sleep. For hours, I'd stare into space. I didn't want to talk to anyone, not even God. I was angry. For days, weeks and months, I binge-watched episodes of TLC's "A Baby Story" and cried. Why did I do that? It wasn't good for my mood or mind.

GOD WOULD USE THE PAIN

All I could see back then was how devastating and cruel it felt. I couldn't think ahead to the future. It didn't occur to me that someday, God would use the pain I'd gone through as a ministry tool for other women who had miscarried also.

In the Kingdom of God, no pain is wasted. No tear is purposeless. Teardrops water the soil of destiny. In due time, beautiful things spring forth from the ground of heartbreak. I am thankful that I can compassionately and empathetically offer comfort to women feeling that hurt.

I know what it is.

Trials are incredible trainers. They teach you all sorts of things: bedside manner; what to say and what not say; when to be silent and when to speak; how to pick up the phone, visit, or help out someone in bad shape when others would avoid them.

If you're in the midst of a major negative life-shift, this is your training ground. You may not fully know why you're going through it, but this moment is not for you or about you. It is about the greater good.

It is about the advancement of God's Kingdom.

It is about you helping someone else after you come through. It is about you sharing your testimony of freedom through Christ. It is about making you an effective witness to the saving, life-giving, sustaining, and supernatural power of God.

My stint with illness took me through some elite-level training. Without it, I would not be able to relate to the frustration, hopelessness and desperation of those that suffer for an extended time period.

Now I can identify with the chronically ill. I am moved to compassionate action when the plight of the helpless is brought to my attention.

That's because, I, too, was helpless. And since God showed mercy, by extending a helping hand to me, I am on a mission to do the same for others.

It's not about me. It never was and it never will be.

A prayer for you: *God, they don't understand why. Aside from the hardship, the uncertainty of it all makes times like these feel even harder. They don't know what You're doing.*

They can't see the purpose of this suffering season. From the looks of things, it will never change. Satan wants them to feel stuck in a rut and victimized by life, when they are already victorious through Christ.

But I pray Ephesians 3:16 over their life today, that from Your glorious, unlimited resources, You will empower them with inner strength through Your Spirit. Until the revelation of Your purpose fully unfolds, may they walk by faith and not by sight.

Please fortify their faith and encourage them to know that weeping may endure for a night, but joy does come in the morning.

In Jesus' name, Amen.

PHASE FOUR

SELFISHNESS
Come out of the You-niverse.

In October 2017, I was invited to Memphis, Tennessee to visit St. Jude Children's Research Hospital that pioneers research and treatments for kids with cancer. My husband Kenya and I attended the annual "Celebration of Hope" weekend, and it was an eye-opening experience.

For the first time, we toured the facilities and learned about how the hospital makes sure the patients' families don't incur any costs for treatment. After leaving, I began raising awareness of St. Jude and encouraging colleagues, family and ministry supporters to donate. You can learn more by visiting www.StJude.org.

When I left, I kept thinking about the fact that, although survival rates are increasing, more can be done. Childhood cancer and pediatric sickle cell disease still tear through tiny bodies, fragment homes, and create devastating realities no loving mom or dad wants to live through.

I WASN'T THE ONLY ONE

When I was going through my health crisis, I felt like I was the only one suffering greatly, and that it would never end, but that's the myth of pain. I wasn't the only one; there are others that fight much fiercer battles.

Parents bury children. Husbands bury wives. My own soulmate would have been planning my home-going service had it not been for divine intervention. I realize there are plenty of people every day that put up a fight against cancer, autoimmune diseases and various other maladies, and lose. When they transition, they often aren't ready to go. Before breathing their last breath, they do everything they can to extend life. They pray not to leave loved ones behind.

Parents' hearts shatter in a million pieces at the thought of not seeing their babies grow up, graduate, get married and produce grandchildren. The infirmed often desire longevity, but don't get it. Just as my loved ones and friends did, their loved ones and friends also form prayer circles, and intercede. Yet, the family member, friend, or colleague, for whom they pray, still passes on.

When I was in the throes of sickness, I didn't think about that. All I could see was my own health woes. But I wasn't the only one in an unfortunate situation. Still and all, I was only focused on myself. I was preoccupied with my issues. I didn't have as keen of an awareness as I do now of how many other women, men, children and families are anguishing.

ME-VILLE

I was engrossed in planning my Woe Is Me bash, sponsored by Why Me, Inc.

The party was taking place on Unfairness Road in the town of Me-Ville, the place I relocated to when my health problems started popping up. Prior to becoming chronically ill, I had rejected multiple invites to take up residence on Unfairness Road.

But as I grew jaded and tired of waiting for God to change my situation, I packed up and moved there.

It conveniently sits in the center of the You-niverse where residents are so concerned with their own problems, they can't see anyone else's. Instead of windows, there are mirrors everywhere in Me-Ville, making it possible for property owners to look at themselves all day, every day.

As part of the lease agreement I signed, I agreed to these terms:

> *Residents of Me-Ville can never be used to bless others because their vision is clouded by their own wants, needs and problems. It is always about them.*

I didn't like those terms and conditions, but, all things considered, I felt it was worth the move anyway.

My dwelling place was on an elevated piece of land, custom-designed to make my issues look bigger than they were. That was premium Me-Ville real estate. That brick house on the mountainous molehill made me feel really special.

Are you living in Me-Ville right now? If so, no judgment. I already told you I'd relocated to one of those grandiose estates. It's true that I don't live there anymore, but I get the appeal.

Why did I move away, you ask? Well, I listened to my counselor, the Holy Spirit. He urged me to pack up and leave, despite all my boxes and belongings being fresh off the moving truck. It's a good thing He didn't let me stay there, because there was a much better place on the other side of town.

"This is where you belong," said the Holy Spirit, pointing toward Selfless Boulevard.

Wow, I could hardly believe I'd be welcomed over there.

It was lovely.

I was told I'd be required to make some changes to my lifestyle, though. I would have to put residents in the neighborhood before myself. I consented to that change, signed the new lease and moved in.

Here's an interesting fact about Selfless Boulevard. There are no mirrors, just windows, in all the houses. It's located in the Kingdom of God and is known for its panoramic views of others' needs and prayer requests, which are on display 24/7. Daily, we have to roll up our sleeves and carry the infirmed and helpless to Jesus, a nice Jewish man and carpenter who helps the needy.

MAKE THE MOVE

Full disclosure: the cost of living on Selfless Boulevard is much higher. You have to sacrifice everything to stay here. But I've been over here a while now and I must say, the experience is quite wonderful.

I encourage you to make the move. It is richly rewarding. I live near some pretty amazing people, too.

Bishop Michael and First Lady Joyce Badger, of Bethesda World Harvest International Church in Buffalo, stay in this neighborhood. After God healed me, they opened their doors for me to share my testimony one Sunday morning. I cried as I shared. It was a full-circle moment for me.

You see, when the Badgers first heard about what was going on with me, Lady J called. She told me she wanted to be a blessing to me and my family. So she went to Sam's Club and bought hundreds of dollars in groceries to our home; the bags were full of delicious goodies for the Hobbs children, since I was unable to prepare meals.

She didn't stay long. She softly prayed, encouraged me, and left.

Lady J and Bishop Badger have been such a great blessing—both during and after my ordeal. They have quietly blessed my family with no fanfare, and I appreciate them deeply.

Wynetta Hall-McElveen, the incredibly generous soul you'll hear more about later in the book, lives here, too. She cooked meals for our family during my sickness. She came to my home, sat down on the floor, sang worship songs and prayed over me. She even kept on cooking meals for our family after God worked the miracle. Pretty awesome, right?

Though the Badgers are real people and Wynetta is a real person, by now, you have gathered that, Unfairness Road and Selfless Boulevard are not real—at least not in the sense of being physical locations.

They *do*, however, exist in our hearts and minds. And I can tell you from experience, if you want to live a fulfilled life, be Christ-like, and see God's will done through you, steer clear of Unfairness Road. Move to Selfless Boulevard; there's always room.

AN OUTBREAK OF VIOLENCE

"I want a divorce!" I told Kenya, crying. "I'm leaving you as soon as I get better." I could barely talk, walk, or function. How was I going to leave anybody?

When I was saying it, I knew it sounded ludicrous, but I couldn't stop myself from uttering those words. My poor husband just sat there, befuddled, as the bizarre statements streamed out of my mouth. "I'm not happy!" I exclaimed.

The more I talked, the angrier I got. My emotions had a bad case of road rage and were driving me insane. Before I knew it, I was literally fighting Kenya. Yes, you read that right.

There was an outbreak of violence in the Hobbs household caused by none other than me.

I was swinging at my best friend and unsuccessfully trying to kick him. Since I was very feeble, sluggish and slow, I didn't have the ability to hurt him, but I sure tried.

I'm not proud of my drug-fueled outburst, but I must tell you the whole truth, not just the pretty parts. The side effects of one of my 13 medications had pushed me over the edge one night. My altered mental state had me thinking I was the Heavyweight Champion of the World and Kenya was my opponent.

Our bedroom turned into a boxing ring. The bell rung and I came out of the corner throwing haymakers.

When I look back on it, I can hardly believe this happened. But, by this time, specialists had identified my two autoimmune diseases. They were in the process of figuring out just the right combination of pills to control my symptoms. I was on a newly prescribed drug called Gabapentin; it helped to ease my severe nerve pain.

Among its many side effects were depression, suicidal thoughts, aggressive or violent behavior. Kenya and I noted this when learning about the drug, but were initially dismissive of the information. At that point, the neuropathic pain was so keen, I would do anything to make it stop. Besides, I was so full of prescriptions, one more pill seemed harmless, but it wasn't.

While I had dealt with uncomfortable side effects before, they were relatively minor. The worst ones, for me, were diarrhea, nausea, wooziness, headaches, drowsiness, increase or loss of appetite. I'd never dealt with psychosis, which is what Gabapentin caused.

When I first started taking it, I noticed troublesome changes. My temper was shorter. I felt moodier and more irritable. I was angrier; everything upset me. Fibromyalgia already caused mood issues, so I didn't need any help being emotionally unstable. After I swallowed each dosage, if it didn't make me mad at the world, I was severely depressed.

Prior to the day I snapped, I felt like a ticking time bomb. And, sure enough, one evening, without warning, the Gabapentin pushed my detonator. I exploded. Boy, was it ugly! I was determined to knock Kenya out. I grabbed any object I could and tried to fling it at him. My coordination was a slight notch above a newborn baby trying to clench a rattle for the first time.

Thank God I was powerless. I am grateful that I was physically impaired. Who knows what would have happened if I had been at full strength? I could have seriously injured Kenya.

Needless to say, he called my doctor and got me taken off that prescription right away. I was shamefaced and excessively apologetic after I got the Gabapentin out of my system.

DIDN'T I DESERVE A PITY PARTY?

That was the first time I'd ever been in an altered mental state like that. The fact that something could override my will and control me without my consent was pretty scary.

I was in a real bind.

Drugs or no drugs, my issues weren't going away. My back was against the wall. I had another woe is me moment. Didn't I deserve a pity party?

Though the Lord could have made the hurt stop, He didn't do that for me. I wasn't happy. And confessing God's promises did not anesthetize or lessen the intensity of the throbbing, aching, stabbing sensations.

There was no remedy that doctors could identify. Day in and day out, I was tormented. My soul was weary and longed desperately for relief.

I seemed to have pretty good grounds to be sad if you asked me. But my oldest sister, Cherisse, whom I just call Ree, texted me.

At first, she wanted to just check in and see how I was doing. A while later, she began calling more regularly and chatting with me when I felt up to it.

Ree encouraged me and assured me that God would bring me through. She was so inspirational for me at that time and helped me cancel my pity party.

PULLING ME OUT OF IT

On one particular day, I was feeling especially low and sick when big sis dialed me up. She wasn't calling to shoot the breeze, nor to get the latest health update, but to pray. Ree, who is a conference founder, television host, author, and preacher of the gospel, prayed Heaven down.

The anointing of the Holy Ghost arrested me in my room. Something shifted in the atmosphere. She interceded for me until the grip of depression released its hold. I could feel God pulling me out of it. Strongholds were crumbling and demons were quaking.

Before my prayer service was ever planned, Cherisse prophesied to me that God would heal me at my brother, Bishop Joseph Brinson, Jr.'s church. Upon hearing that word, I received it and planned to go to Covenant of Grace. But I was never well enough to make it.

I didn't know the Lord had a predestined date for my healing, which took place, as God said through her, in Bishop Brinson's sanctuary. How about that? What an amazing God we serve. He used Cherisse to give me a small glimpse of His master plan before unveiling it completely.

On the night of my healing, she was at a church service in Atlanta. A prophetess there ministered to Cherisse and told her God had healed me. My sister was so elated, she danced before the Lord on my behalf.

After the service in was over, Ree said she looked on the Internet and saw posts everywhere about the miracle God worked in my life. Incredible.

Prayer and encouragement sessions with Ree made me want to have a praise party instead of a pity party, even before I was made whole. I canceled my doomsday plans and started rejoicing when she was on the line with me.

She suggested songs for me to listen to and videos to watch. I began feasting on the goodness of the Lord. Worship melodies were my constant companion; I drowned out Satan's whispers with uplifting tunes.

There were many people God used to keep on pulling me out of my pit of despair. My sister Quinny also sent me songs, checked on me daily, counseled and calmed me. My brother Lamond, a gifted musician and composer, created and recorded an instrumental worship track for me. It soothed my spirit as David's harp-playing soothed Saul's in 1 Samuel 16:14-23.

Elder Malcolm Wilson, who was the first person outside of my family to know of my predicament, deposited a powerful word from God into my life. I was scheduled to emcee a musical for his choir, Joshua's Generation, but I was too ill. I wasn't yet ready to let the cat out of the bag about my health, but I had to tell him why I would be forced to cancel my appearance that had already been advertised.

Malcom said my sickness was not unto death, but for God to receive the glory. He was at my prayer service to see the manifestation of the word he spoke over my life.

My brothers Andre, Dion, Donte and Bishop Christopher Brinson prayed, believed and trusted God to do the impossible. They never spoke a word of negativity; just faith.

My brother Joseph Brinson, III, whom I just call Joe-Joe, talked faith to me, no matter what doctors said. One afternoon, he sang an original song to me over the phone that broke me down in tears. It was just what I needed to hear.

His wife, my sister and friend, Patrice, a three-time breast cancer survivor and my shero, talked to me, encouraged me, and asked her prayer group to pray for me in North Carolina. On Christmas, Joe-Joe and Patrice surprised me with a visit. They brought me so much joy.

My sister Shante, mighty prayer warrior that she is, didn't express an ounce of worry. Not only did she pray me through some of my roughest nights all the way from North Carolina, but she agreed to be an intercessor for my prayer service. She and her husband Rafiq made the trip to Buffalo to be there.

The texts, calls and love from all my family members and friends, who are too numerous to name, were such a great help to me.

Though I was afflicted in my body and had plenty down days, they lifted me up. They helped me cancel lots of pity parties and instead, break open my alabaster box and pour my worship on the Lord like oil.

ROCK BOTTOM

As I write this, I find that words fail me. My attempts to articulate the severity of the pain, shocking nature of the circumstances, and the depth of misery I felt, fall short.

How do I convey how difficult and demoralizing it was to go from being strong, always on the go, bubbly and productive, to being bedridden, wearing adult diapers? How do I express the inexpressible sorrow, disillusionment, complexity and cruelty of my situation? Adjectives and phrases suddenly seem to be in short supply.

My quality of life could be summed up in two words: rock bottom.

Down there, I had no long speeches or lengthy prayers. I was doing well just to choke out a raspy, *help me*. I couldn't exert the energy to shout loudly and scream for assistance. Only my anguished soul cried through sealed lips the words of Psalm 22:1 KJV: "My God, my God, why hast thou forsaken me? Why art thou so far from helping me, and from the words of my roaring?"

Feeling forsaken, alone and forgotten, was the worst. This is why writing *God Did It* has been hard. I don't wish to once again tour the dark, murky cave of loneliness and depression. But how ungrateful of me would it be to deprive the world of my testimony because I don't want to *go there.*

That would be selfish.

Moses didn't want to go there, to Egypt (Exodus 4). Jonah didn't want to go there, to Nineveh (Jonah 1:3). Jesus didn't want to go there, to Calvary (Matthew 26:39). But in each case, someone's deliverance was tied to their willingness to go there. Their quality of life took a hit also. Jesus gave up the most. So, sacrificing is the least I can do. It is my reasonable service (Romans 12:1).

Penning this autobiographical nonfiction work has forced me to retrace the faint chalk lines I unsuccessfully tried to erase. I didn't (and still don't) want to relive what God, by His grace, brought me through. I've had to repeatedly tell myself,

Dianna, what you went through is not about you. It is for someone else. Someone needs to know, not just that I *did* make it, but *how* I made it.

It was a hard-fought battle. It wasn't pretty. I took some frontline fire and sustained injuries, but because my weapons of warfare are not carnal, but mighty through God, according 2 Corinthians 10:4, every stronghold had to come down. The enemy could not win.

He hit me with his best shots, and when he did, God was there.

When I hit rock bottom, Jesus, indeed, was the Rock *at* the bottom. The Lord never left me. As bad as my quality of life was for a time, God's presence kept me.

FREAKING OUT

I recall sending a text to Kenya's phone one day when I was having trouble processing that sickness was part of my new reality.

This is the private message he received from his distressed wife:

> *I'm freaking out that I'm sick—that I'm actually sick and can't control it. Today it's freaking me out. I don't know how my quality of life can take such a turn for the worst and I can't do anything to change it. Not understanding this. Sorry. Just needed to vent and get that off my chest today. It all makes life feel really uncertain and scary.*

Kenya wrote back:

> *Take God's word and meditate on these things in Isaiah 41:10: "So do not fear, for I am with you; do not be dismayed, for I am your God. I will strengthen you and help you; I will uphold you with my righteous right hand." Babe, though your hand may be shaky, His is steady. And though your body may be weak, He is strong. And even while you don't understand what's going on, He says, "Trust in Me with all your heart and I will make your path straight." Remember, while you may not know, HE knows all! You're in good hands. Rest in Him.*

What a comforting message he sent back. That day was a particularly bad one.

When Kenya said "though your hand may be shaky," it wasn't metaphorical. I could barely hold my phone steady to send the message because of the hand tremors I was experiencing. The bad case of the shakes, which took over my legs as well, happened several times weekly, for no apparent reason.

There was an invisible assailant holding me hostage. I could feel its grip. My body no longer obeyed me. The signals and commands my brain was sending were getting lost.

My arms, hands, feet, and joints had become uncontrollable. If I said go left, my members went right. I had become a house divided against itself and I could not stand. I could not stand physically.

I also could not stand: being broken; being locked up in my room; feeling like a burden; needing someone to hold me up with each step; the way I was feeling; my diminished quality of life. I could not stand it!

Before reaching out to Kenya that afternoon, I'd had a sort of negative epiphany. It hit me and freaked me out that this wasn't a bad dream. The symptoms weren't going away. I had a frightening new normal. I was in unknown territory, and this trial was going to require a particular fruit of the spirit mentioned in Galatians 5:22: longsuffering.

And suffer long I did. But here I stand. God resurrected me from the ashes. He will resurrect you, too. He has given me a new lease on life. These days, I don't worry so much about my quality of life, but the quality of my relationship with the giver of life.

He is the source of my contentment, peace and victory. My relationship with Him is my greatest joy, and my chief desire is to selflessly serve Him by tirelessly serving others.

I WEPT BITTERLY

Prior to the discovery that autoimmune diseases were attacking my eyes, when I was diagnosed with Glaucoma in 2015, I thought it was an isolated incident. I would later discover that it was symptomatic of the underlying causes that set off a chain of events within.

Since I didn't know that this was simply a link in that chain of symptoms caused by a bigger issue, I felt blindsided by the news that I'd be blind within five years.

I wept bitterly upon hearing that.

Glaucoma is called the "sneak thief of sight" because it frequently goes undetected, making it a leading cause of blindness.

That thief snuck up on me silently and had already stolen a good portion of my vision before it was detected.

The discovery phase started at LensCrafters in a local mall. I had been having trouble with blurry vision, so I got an eye exam. The optometrist told me I was nearsighted and gave me a written prescription for eyeglasses. I picked out frames I liked, paid the cost, and thought that was it.

Not exactly.

The friendly eye doctor told me he spotted something troubling on my films and I needed to see a specialist.

"Okay," I said, slowly and confusedly, but not thinking too much of it. I made an appointment with an ophthalmologist, who examined the films and tested my eyes.

The news I got back was startling.

My Intraocular pressure (IOP), the fluid pressure inside my eye, was so high, it had done major irreversible damage. My Glaucoma had progressed to the degree that I could expect to lose my sense of sight. I was informed matter-of-factly that there was no way I could save my vision.

"I need to be honest with you," the specialist said. "Within the next five years, you will be blind."

Time stopped. I squirmed in my seat. I asked if he was for real. I didn't know what else to say. "You can't be serious," I blurted.

"I am," he said, standing his ground.

I must have asked him some variation of the same question ten different ways: *Am I really going to be blind in five years?* I needed to make sure my ears were hearing him correctly.

Each time, the answer he offered was the same: I was *definitely* going to be without vision. Nothing I proposed could fix it. Vitamin A wouldn't help, no matter how many carrots I ate.

No drops, pills, or procedures could reverse the damage.

He elaborated and stressed that the five-year rough estimate was a generous one. I could go blind in *less* time. This was the top specialist in the region talking, mind you.

There are only three eye specialists in Western New York, and he trained the other two.

So much for wanting a second opinion.

When I phoned my friend Cassandra Elliott, whom I mentioned earlier, I was distraught. Thus, the bitter weeping.

GOD ALWAYS HAS THE FINAL SAY

I affectionately call Cassandra, PC, which is short for Pastor Cassandra. She is an award-winning worship pastor in North Carolina and a powerful prayer warrior.

Before getting her on the phone, I was sitting alone in the parking lot behind my big black glasses they made me wear upon leaving. The protective eyewear blocked the sun. Since I had just had a special procedure done, my eyes could not be exposed to its bright rays for a few hours. That meant I couldn't drive.

Just great.

I wasn't expecting such an intense testing process, not naturally or spiritually. I had come alone. Now that I needed a chauffeur, I had to wait for Kenya. For several minutes, I sat there, locked inside my car, having a woe is me party.

I was a wreck. I thought of what this diagnosis meant. Blindness was unfathomable, the news I'd absorbed was unfavorable, and I was inconsolable.

By the time I got on the line with PC, I was sniffling and struggling to articulate the report of the doctor. Ideally, I would have hidden my sadness, but I was too devastated to fake like I wasn't.

Thank God for a spiritually-sensitive friend. She made it her business to speak only the report of the Lord. She could have started mourning with me over what the chief eye specialist said my outcome would be. But PC reminded me that God always has the final say.

From thousands of miles away, she began praying for this shaken up Buffalo girl. Without asking any questions or trying to get the juicy details, she simply joined her faith with mine. She interceded with power and authority.

When she addressed God, she didn't ask Him to heal me just so I could see for the rest of my days. She asked the Lord to deliver me for the sake of the call, which means for the purpose of fulfilling my ministry assignment on earth.

We all have a divine calling, a purpose, and a specific role to fulfill for the benefit of the Kingdom. PC's focus was on mine.

SHIFTING MY PERSPECTIVE

"You know Dianna needs her eyes to do Your work," she said in her impassioned plea to God. With just those words alone, she shifted my perspective to my calling. I was now thinking about ministry and how my eyesight is needed to continue reaching souls all over the world.

It wasn't just about wanting to be whole for the sake of being whole, but for the sake of the call.

PC didn't simply request that God heal my eyes, but she decreed and declared that He would give me *new eyes*. By the time she finished, I felt a weight lift off of me. I could feel the presence of God all over me. Even though nothing in my circumstances was noticeably different, I felt brand new. Shifting my perspective to my purpose unburdened me, even before God shifted my situation.

I needed PC that day.

Hear me out on this: when you get blindsided by life, you need people like PC who will pray you through and keep your mind elevated. Weak-hearted ones will start weeping, panicking and mourning like the folks did in Matthew 9:18-25.

Do you remember when the 12-year-old daughter of a man named Jairus fell sick and died, and the mourners came over to the house? There was a heavy atmosphere of sorrow. I can imagine the screams and muffled sobs. In my mind's eye, I can see relatives and close friends holding onto each other, talking about what a shame it was that this child was gone so soon.

When Jesus stepped into the house, He didn't join in with the mourners. Rather, He declared that the damsel wasn't dead, but sleeping. Unlike those around Him, He didn't base His evaluation of the situation on what was apparent to the eye. To those that couldn't get past the obvious, what Jesus said sounded like utter foolishness and folly.

The non-believers scoffed at Him. The wailers wiped away their crocodile tears and started mocking the Master instead.

They were sure the miracle-worker, whose reputation for healing preceded Him, had, this time, lost His mind for sure.

I love Jesus's response to their unbelief. He wouldn't let them dwell there. He put everybody out that was carnally-minded. PC kicked carnality out of the car that day and said we're making a petition *for the sake of the call.* Months later, her petitions and declarations manifested in a monumental way.

SOMETHING HAD CHANGED

When I revisited the ophthalmologist after using the drops he prescribed, something supernatural happened. Not only had my intraocular pressure normalized, but the specialist had to change the prognosis.

During my reexamination, I could tell he was unsettled.

As he peered into my eyes, magnifying them through the lenses of his big old fancy, expensive, powerful machine, it was obvious something had changed.

He flipped through my file in puzzlement. After some head-scratching moments passed, he told me my eyes didn't only look better, but, he said —and I quote— "It looks almost like you have *new eyes.*"

I could have run around the halls of the office! What Cassandra decreed and declared by faith is what the specialist confirmed verbatim. God had given me *new eyes.* That grim prognosis changed.

Before that, he told me I needed to have surgery right away. Furthermore, even if I did have the operation, the damage could not be reversed; but God bypassed the natural surgeon and operated on my eyes Himself.

That miracle God worked on my eyes started with a two-person prayer service in a car. Matthew 18:20 NASB is true, which says, "For where two or three have gathered together in My name, I am there in their midst."

PC expelled doubt and spoke faith into the atmosphere. We touched and agreed, for the sake of the call, and God showed up.

He will show up in your life also. But first, He wants you to realize that your miracle, breakthrough, increase, provision and every good and perfect gift is for His glory. When you trade selfishness for selflessness and give your life for the sake of the call, He will shower you with blessings and favor. You'll have so many testimonies of your own to point to and declare, *God did it!*

COME OUT OF HIDING

What I was going through sent shockwaves throughout the faith community. People near and far, who are familiar with the ministry God has given me, were astonished to hear of my misfortune. As you well know by now, none of this was ever supposed to get out. I had privatized my pain and planned to keep it that way.

How selfish of me to deprive others who loved me and would be eager to stand in faith with me of the opportunity to pray. I needed to come out of hiding.

Nonetheless, I was in Me-Ville. I was not interested in an awareness campaign to broadcast the details of my sad situation. But how could worldwide warriors unify under the banner of prayer if no one rallied them?

Privately, I had already experienced the overwhelming power of focused, specific, faith-filled, fervent prayer.

One day, my brother, Bishop Joseph Brinson, Jr., reached out to me via phone. I was happy to hear from him and not surprised that he had a word from the Lord to release. The prophetic anointing on his life is clear and undeniable. His gift has touched so many across the nation.

When he phoned me, he didn't ask me what was wrong. He didn't question me about my symptoms. He *told me* what my symptoms were, calling some things out by name that no one was aware of but me, Kenya, my doctors, and of course, God. My brother wasn't familiar with the details of my health case. But the Lord, the great revealer of secrets, told him. Then Bishop spoke to those conditions and commanded them to loose me.

While we were talking, pain left. That swimming feeling in my head disappeared. By the time he hung up, God had given me some welcome relief. Though the challenges were numerous, a few of the battles I was fighting before Bishop agreed with me, were no longer issues following our telephone prayer meeting. Those things never plagued me again.

I know prayer works, which is why selfishly closing myself off from public prayer wasn't exercising wisdom. I was being carnal and thinking only about what made me comfortable. That's what kept me from coming out of hiding.

Since I live my life publicly and communicate regularly through blogs, vlogs, podcasts, social media posts, newsletters, and in-person appearances, going off the radar left those who are connected to me through some or all of those channels, concerned.

They were already reaching out to our ministry staff constantly. Phones were ringing. Email inboxes were full. Something needed to be said.

But there was radio silence, at least for a while, because I was making it personal, when all along it was *spiritual*. I needed to hurry up and move flesh out of the way.

I was worried about not wanting to be made a public spectacle when God wanted to work a public miracle. My desire for comfort was clashing with His desire for glory.

The attack of the enemy was intensifying. I had walked into the roaring lion's lair and he had a plan to devour me. Before God dropped it in my spirit, I wasn't aware that another prayer service—a much larger one than the car session I had with PC—would be necessary.

My dear friend Cassandra would be there, too, along with many other powerful women of God.

I STOPPED BEING SELFISH

Before that memorable March 2017 date-with-destiny arrived, I stopped being selfish and gave my team permission to open up about my ordeal.

Once the news of my illness was finally revealed to the public, I was moved by the overwhelming amount of love, prayer and support I received. What was I ever afraid for?

Initially, I had been fighting Satan with a small army of in-the-know comrades. When I told my mother, she put the whole family on notice—as well as some of her friends, and ministry leaders she believed could get a prayer through. When my ministry staff put the word out, however, that's when the floodgates opened, and a mighty army of believers unleashed righteous fury on the enemy.

It was awesome. I felt strengthened and uplifted. There were gifts, cards, care packages, books, Bibles, and all kinds of things to motivate and comfort me, both naturally *and* spiritually. God used folks I knew and ones I didn't to usher in His presence, bless me, uphold me, and plant seeds of faith in the soil of my heart.

When I stopped being selfish, I saw how selfless others were and my world was rocked in the best way.

DON'T MAKE THIS ALL ABOUT YOU

Coming out of Me-Ville resulted in something far more beautiful than I could have conceived. When I got over myself, God sent me a global team of Holy Ghost-filled prayer warriors. Folks from different time zones, races, ethnicities, cultures and creeds came together.

They weren't afraid to boldly ask God to move in my favor. As shocking as the news of my physical deterioration was, they believed by God's power I would rise again. Spiritually-minded praying women and men asked the Lord for help. They fervently requested that He would lift me up and make me a testimony of His greatness.

Well, God did it, but not until after I stopped hiding naturally and opted for a life that is spiritually "hidden with Christ in God" (Colossians 3:3). He is my hiding place; under the shadow of His wings I find safety. He is my refuge. I now know I don't have to slip into self-preservation mode, for He will preserve me in times of sorrow, trouble and distress.

Friend, the Lord is your preserver and keeper, too.

He is your shelter. He is your guide. If you want to tap into all He is and what He is able to do, come out of the You-niverse and get lost in *His* will. Don't make this all about you.

Realize that He's up to something far more beautiful, masterful and powerful than you could ever orchestrate on your own.

A prayer for you: God, in lack and in plenty; in sickness and in wellness; in hard times and in good times; in all circumstances, let them seek after Your will and not their own.

You have allowed this test as a way to develop their character. You are teaching them to look beyond themselves and see the greater purpose in their struggle. It is for the glory of Your name.

The enemy wants to make them self-focused so that they will lose sight of their divine assignment. But I thank You for refocusing them today and getting them ready for the great exploits they will do for Your Kingdom.

Reassure them that, when they come through this test, they will be blessed above measure because You can trust them to be a blessing.

In Jesus' name, Amen.

PHASE FIVE

DEFEATED

Satan is already defeated, but his tactic is to convince you that you are.

―∞✟∞―

I was up against a formidable opponent and it seemed like defeat was inevitable. It looked that way for a man named Gideon in the Bible; the Lord laid it on my heart to begin this phase with his story.

When the Angel of the Lord addressed Gideon as a "mighty man of valor" and told him God was going to use him to save Israel out of the hand of the Midianites in Judges 6, he could hardly believe it.

Gideon, whose name means "cutter" or "cutter of trees," was ordinary in every sense of the word. His family wasn't esteemed. He was a coward. And yet, God called him.

Feeling small and unworthy, and hiding out from the enemy, Gideon replied, "O my Lord, how can I save Israel? Indeed my clan is the weakest in Manasseh, and I am the least in my father's house" (Judges 6:15 NKJV).

FOCUS ON GOD'S BIGNESS

Do you see what Gideon did? He focused on his smallness, instead of God's bigness. He zoned in on his own weakness, instead of God's strength. We make that mistake sometimes, too.

He let his lack of confidence fool him into thinking he didn't hold a high enough position to be triumphant. Gideon thought he couldn't be used by God to defeat the enemy, because he was too defeated in his mindset to see that, with God, all things are possible (Matthew 19:26).

But there is nothing too hard for the Lord. Whoever you are, wherever you come from, whatever disadvantages you may be dealing with, God's plan for your life will come full circle.

As I told you before, He levels the playing field. So focus on His bigness, not your own smallness or perceived inadequacies.

No one and nothing can stop Him from blessing you, using you, elevating you, increasing you, delivering you, working a miracle for you, and making you an example of the amazing things His power can do.

HE IS YET FAITHFUL

Gideon, one of the most fearful judges of Israel, was so down on himself and had such poor self-image, that he could not wrap his mind around the fact that God commanded little old him to save the nation.

You know what Gideon did?

He asked God for several signs to convince him of the validity of the divine call according to Judges 6:36-40. God was merciful enough to prove Himself, even though He was by no means obligated to do so.

Aren't you grateful for God's grace, and how He has compassion on us despite our shortcomings?

When we are faithless, He is yet faithful. He's faithful to deliver.

When it was all said and done, Gideon accepted his calling, only to have God reduce his army of 32,000 men to 300. In the natural, this was a recipe for defeat—especially against the cruel and seemingly invincible Midianites.

They had been bullying the Israelites for quite some time. Everyone was terrified of these men God used to judge the wrongdoing of His chosen people. But when time came for God to deliver Israel, He didn't need a whole lot to do it.

Gideon, with only those chosen 300, went up against the Midianites. Funny thing is, after being scared and hesitant, he didn't have to do much except make some noise!

The Israelites blew rams' horns, shouted, broke jars, and just like that, sent the enemy running.

In an instant, the battle was over and the victory was won. The fight was already fixed. All Gideon and his army had to do was show up, and God did the rest.

If we can remember that it is God's power that puts the enemy on the run, we won't be so quick to become intimidated by the attacks against us. If we could recall that God is faithful to deliver us, no matter how it looks, we wouldn't panic so easily.

As sick as I was, had I kept God's faithfulness and bigness constantly on my mind, would I have panicked so easily? Of course not. But my humanness got the best of me sometimes. I let Satan get in my ear and whisper lies.

You don't have to falter in this area. Satan is already defeated because God's power is greater than what's coming against you. You can rest in the midst of the storm.

GOD CHOSE 50

After being pounded relentlessly by complicated issues for months, I was closer than ever to my shift. Satan had worked tirelessly to convince me I was defeated, when really, he was defeated all along.

God's weapon of choice against him was intercessory prayer.

The Lord told me to call valiant warriors in the Kingdom and ask the women of God to pray. Gideon had 300 soldiers. In my case, God chose 50 intercessors.

He made me aware that the number of women He selected specifically related to the symbolism of the 50th year.

In scripture, according to Leviticus 25, the 50th year is known biblically as "The Year of Jubilee," when liberty was proclaimed throughout the land. In the Old Testament, during Jubilee, land would be returned to its rightful owner and slaves would be freed from the bonds of servitude.

I was about to get free. It had been long enough.

On that special night, God promised me that, as 50 prayer warriors touched and agreed, submitted to the assignment and interceded, strongholds would be broken, shackles would be loosed, and spiritual Jubilee would take place.

God would release healing, restoration, deliverance and renewal. His glory would fall. He would restore what was lost, just as He declared in Joel 2:25.

I knew this was a divinely-inspired vision and I had better move. I felt like I was floundering in the waters of the unknown, but I refused to get back in the boat.

I PUT SOME FEET ON MY FAITH

I walked on water at His beckoning, not because I was some giant in the faith, but because I trusted in the One who called me. I didn't have all the details or answers, but I put some feet on my faith. I trusted God to order the steps I took and lead me to my miracle.

Clear as the vision was, I was *unclear* about how to implement it. I was too feeble in my body to do it alone. Yet, after God spoke it to me, I attempted to make calls with my raspy voice.

My first call was to Pastor Valerie Foye of Greater Apostolic House of Prayer in Buffalo. She later told me that hearing my voice scared her. That's how bad I sounded!

But I was willing to do whatever it took to honor God's command. I sensed He was up to something and I didn't want to miss out on whatever it was.

My sweet sister-in-law, Lady Bertha Brinson, agreed to let me hold the prayer service at Covenant of Grace Fellowship International, the church she leads alongside my brother, Bishop Joseph Brinson, Jr. in Niagara Falls, New York.

I had the date. I had the venue. I had the vision. Now I needed a fellow visionary to take the reins and pull it together.

That's when a family member told me a local worship leader, recording artist and longtime friend, Wynetta Hall McElveen, my neighbor on Selfless Boulevard (Remember her?), was looking for me. When we connected, Wynetta was crying on the phone, telling me about the vision God gave her.

"We have to have a prayer service for you," she said.

I was shocked. My jaw dropped. He gave her the same directives He'd given me. Her assignment was my assignment, which was all the confirmation I needed. She had been sent to me.

See what putting some feet on your faith will do? When you start moving in the direction of what God said by faith, He will open the floodgates of favor and cause blessings to overwhelm you.

I broke down in tears, overcome with emotion. I had been concerned about the logistics and how it would get done. Meanwhile, God already had the plan, and the person to implement it, in place. He was just testing me.

THEY BELIEVED THE WORD OF GOD

The prayer warriors were handpicked from various denominations. Some I knew well, others I didn't know at all. There were some names God gave me specifically and others the planning team added.

Having a close relationship with me was not a prerequisite. Having a close relationship with God was. The intercessors couldn't be fearful or skeptical. They were called to combat the enemy and remind him of his place: under our feet.

Only those anointed to war in the spirit until a shift took place in the earth realm were tapped. They had to possess the stubbornness of Jacob in Genesis 32, when he wrestled with an angel all night long. He refused to let go until he got his blessing.

Our troop of 50 was ready for battle. They repudiated the enemy's false claims that I would be in that predicament forever.

They believed the word of God.

They prayed in faith and the Lord did the rest. He moved that mountain of affliction and set me free.

Satan, the defeated one, that God allowed to torment and buffet me for a season, got his permission slip taken back. His access to me and my body was cut off. He tried to kill me, but God preserved me. Now I am free.

Perhaps you need to be set free. You might be staring at a mountain that needs moving. You could be going through a shocking ordeal. You may be saying, *I never imagined my life would be this way.* You didn't think it would come to this. Where you are looks nothing like the awesome place you envisioned you would be.

The enemy wants you to feel defeated, but you're not. He is. You're a victor.

God is telling you through the pages of *God Did It* that there is a great plan for your deliverance. There is more for you than what you are now witnessing. Lift up your head. Do what Hebrews 12:2 tells you and fix your eyes on Jesus. He is the author and finisher of your faith. Your situation may have taken you by surprise, but the Lord knew you would be where you are before you got here.

And He already mapped out your escape route from trouble.

NO STRANGERS TO THE SUPERNATURAL

I had seen God do the impossible before. While I was carrying our eldest son, Kedar, the ultrasound technician discovered a fetal abdominal tumor during a routine sonogram.

Doctors confirmed the find.

He had a mass covering 50 percent of his stomach. I was notified that surgery would have to be performed right after delivery. I was broken up about it. I gathered family together. We fasted and prayed. When Kedar was born, the tumor, amazingly, had disappeared.

Our youngest daughter, Kaiah, was born without her uvula— that soft pink flesh that dangles in the back of the mouth. There was nothing there but a gaping hole. She had a hard time swallowing without choking; I was told that its nonexistence would negatively impact her speech and she'd have issues for the rest of her life.

Again, we prayed.

When we visited the pediatrician, she was startled after shining a light in Kaiah's mouth. Our baby daughter's uvula had grown in. The physician told me she had never seen anything like that in all her decades of practicing medicine.

"It's a creative miracle!" she said.

My siblings and I are no strangers to the supernatural.

We have seen God's glorious works in the lives of others. As a child traveling across the nation with my father, an evangelist and gospel preacher, I have seen demons expelled, the lame walk, cancers cured, blinded eyes opened, and countless souls saved.

For me, the supernatural is not some bizarre phenomenon. It isn't a phony, contrived scheme to lace the pockets of greedy televangelists, or heretical teachers posing as God's emissaries.

I have seen God work. I have heard rich and powerful testimonies. I never doubted the veracity of the claims of those who had been healed and delivered at the hands of Jesus. I knew He could do the same for me, and yet, I felt defeated.

HOW COULD THAT BE?

How could I know with such confident conviction that God is a miracle-worker and still struggle with feelings of defeat?

How could that be?

I was aware that Jesus is still able to recover the sight of the blind as He did in the case of Bartimaeus (Mark 10:46-52).

I knew He was yet delivering those bound for a long time, as He did with the man at the Pool of Bethesda after a 38-year health crisis (John 5).

But I had reached my breaking point. That's how I ended up struggling. My body was weakening and so was my will to go on. Satan kicked me while I was down one too many times, and dumped a pile of bricks on me to boot. He shamed me for the state I was in. He told me I was worthless and would never rise again.

Satan didn't want me to remember that Colossians 2:15 tells me Jesus had already "disarmed the spiritual rulers and authorities. He shamed them publicly by his victory over them on the cross."

Because of the completed work of Christ, that old rascal was defeated at Calvary. Notwithstanding, Satan is a pretty convincing liar. He points out unfavorable circumstances and introduces them as corroborating evidence of our supposedly inevitable demise.

But as I have said multiple times in this book, the Lamb of God, Jesus Christ, has secured victory on our behalf, despite the odds stacked against us.

And by His stripes, as Isaiah 53:5 says, we are healed.

MY BODY WAVED THE WHITE FLAG

Feelings of defeat grew more intense once I was admitted to Roswell Park Cancer Institute.

My body had waved the white flag of surrender and I needed around-the-clock care. With my bodily functions severely impaired, teams of specialists surrounded my bed, asked questions, examined me, ran tests and pumped me full of potent drugs to keep me going.

I laid in bed for days with the shades drawn in the darkened private suite at the hospital. No television. No book. No food. Just sleep. And pain-numbing narcotics.

I was in a drugged-induced haze, stirring only when breakthrough pain reminded me it was time for another dose. Kenya sat quietly in a recliner next to my bed, holding my hand through the night.

Kenya shared with me a memory of that hospitalization period. Whenever I'd gain consciousness in short spurts, he said, I'd smile through my pain, say "I love you" and then go back out.

I don't remember a lot of things, but I *do* recollect how his thumb went back and forth across my fingers. I can call to mind the soothing nature of his gentle caress.

"That's so sweet," I'd whisper when I'd awaken, and ask, "You've been sitting here all this time holding my hand?"

I thought to myself, *He must be bored. His body must be hurting. He has to be tired.* But Kenya was content as long as he could comfort me with his presence. I was thankful, but I felt guilty.

I viewed myself as burdensome and useless. That marauding thief, Satan, had stolen away my confidence and robbed me of the belief that I was any good to anyone. I had broken down mentally and physically.

I couldn't fulfill my wifely duties. I wasn't able to cook or clean. I was debilitated and sickly, and no longer able to take care of my family.

I felt as if the diseases had finally defeated me. They had beaten my body into submission. Every nerve, muscle, joint and organ surrendered.

My dignity was gone as I was in the hospital, stripped naked and rolled over by a group of nurses looking for bed sores. With gloved hands, they checked every crevice and orifice, apologizing and saying, "We know this is uncomfortable."

Uncomfortable was the understatement of understatements. They were doing their jobs with great care, sensitivity and gentleness. So my humiliation was no fault of theirs. Being totally exposed left me feeling like a cold slab of meat on a table.

I was seen by all, but not truly visible to anyone, except Kenya. I was one of many patients. My body parts were canvases that professionals scanned for signs, symptoms and indicators.

I'd lost my personhood.

I was just a subject. A case study. A problem to be solved. I was just there, barely existing, waiting for my next shot of whatever to make it through another day.

I NEEDED DIVINE RELEASE

The procedures were so impersonal. With all the staff's niceness and attentiveness, I still was ashamed, especially when I soiled myself, and a nurse had to clean it up.

"It's okay, honey," she would say. "That's what I'm here for."

Whenever I'd have an accident, no matter how many times it happened, I'd instinctively say, "I'm so sorry."

"No, don't apologize. That's okay," my nurse would reiterate, doing her best to protect my pride. But I never got used to the idea of needing care like an infant that had to be changed, fed, clothed, washed and put to sleep.

While hospitalized, part of me was happy for the bowel release, despite the embarrassment. My intestinal system had quit functioning for the most part. Feces had backed up and liquefied inside me, and was pushing upward, making it hard to breathe. My bodily wastes had nowhere to go. My situation was critical.

Before I was able to move my bowels, Kenya and I came up with a light-hearted way of requesting prayer specifically for my intestinal issues. "Pray poop prayers," Kenya told everyone. "We need a divine release!"

John 14:14 says, "You may ask me for anything in my name, and I will do it." For me, that "anything" was the ability to defecate.

One night, before being allowed to go home, I woke up. Kenya had dropped off to sleep with his phone in his lap and my palm in his. All was quiet, but my spirit was restless.

It was time to pray. I warred against that defeated spirit. I commanded Satan to take his hands off of me—mind and body. I spoke the word of God in the slightest whisper. I strongly believed I would get my divine release.

For several minutes, a clarity not of this earth came over me. It broke through the side effects of the drugs that usually kept my brain foggy.

Though I was hooked up to those machines, with cords and tubes hanging everywhere, my hookup with God overrode all the other stuff. I could sense His presence in my room. Tears dropped out of my eyes and pooled in my ears. I didn't have physical strength to move or lift my hands, but God lifted my spirit.

I felt His anointing.

I asked the Lord to release me from the grip of disease and death and restore me back to health. The answer to that prayer didn't fully manifest until the following year. But within days, I got my, ahem, divine release.

God unblocked me … temporarily.

A BAD SIGN

When discharge day came, I was so happy. Going home meant I could finally rest in my own bed. Just the thought of it made me smile. I was a little scared, too. The substances that had been pumping through my veins by way of IV were stopped. I had to see how I'd do on my own.

Would I wind up right back in the hospital again? Would my body go through the same cycle that alarmed the overnight care staff at Roswell's Assessment and Treatment Center, and caused them to admit me in the first place?

The way I wound up at Roswell after midnight was unexpected. I'd had a colonoscopy and endoscopy done. Right before my colonoscopy, the surgeon let me know he had identified what looked like a tumor on my films. "I've been doing this a long time and I am pretty certain of what I see," he told me. His blunt delivery of the truth, he said, was to get me ready for the inevitable.

I swallowed hard. I wanted to be strong, but hearing that colon cancer was more than likely the source of my bowel issues, messed me up. The whole thing was already upsetting, but his words were doubly troubling because I thought I was out of the woods.

You see, the night before, when I landed in the ER because of an obstruction in my small intestine, I had been warned that the narrowing doctor's saw was a bad sign.

But, after I prayed, my blood levels regulated and the medical team reexamined me. They told me they could no longer see the issue in my small intestine that had them worried before. Everything looked good. As you might imagine, I was on a high. I was excited. Despite being very ill and fatigued, I was optimistic.

That's why, when the surgeon the following day at Roswell overturned that good report, it was a deflating moment. My helium balloon of joy withered and fell to the floor. With a lump in my throat, I looked over at Kenya. He peered into my eyes and reassured me that God was with me.

Since I was dehydrated and in bad shape, nurse after nurse struggled to find a vein through which anesthesia could be administered for my procedure. But all my veins were collapsed. So was my confidence. I was ice cold and rundown. I had already been through so much.

They called for a veteran anesthesiologist to help out. The tall brunette did her best to find a vein, but ended up bruising my arm terribly. I now had a swollen, sore, battered arm.

SOMEBODY UP THERE IS LOOKING OUT FOR YOU

It was time to call Ken. Thank God he came rushing down to my floor. First, he put me in this odd blowup suit that inflated itself with heat. It was designed to warm up cold patients like me and get some blood flowing. He thought increasing my body temperature would help. Next, he examined my arms and hands, softly pressing on veins and tracing them with his pointer finger.

After some time passed, Ken finally identified a tiny vein in my hand. He warned me that inserting the needle might hurt. I held my breath. After he rubbed the area with an alcohol pad, he tightly gripped the smallest needle he could get his hands on.

Ken directed the tip at my skin and said, "Ready?"

I wasn't, but I had to be.

The initial sharp prick was intense. It burned. Then that burning turned into persistent throbbing. He was right. It hurt. I made sure I didn't move a muscle, though. After some tense moments, the needle was in and I exhaled.

Ken said, "Somebody up there is looking out for you."

That "somebody" was God.

He smiled and added, "I don't ever want to see you back here again."

That made two of us!

When the colonoscopy was over, nurses woke me up. I had made it through okay would have to wait for the full results. I thought the worst was over and looked forward to going back to the house, curling up under my quilt and sleeping off the drugs. I wasn't expecting to have post-procedure complications.

Whenever I tried to move my bowels, it felt like glass shards were cutting me, or a thousand needles were poking me. Why was I feeling faint? Why was my heart beating so fast? Why did my body feel like I had been placed in a freezer, but I was sweating? What was all this heaviness in my abdomen? How come I couldn't stand up straight without extreme pain? Why couldn't I pass stool? And why was the toilet bowl full of rich, red blood?

Wait.

What?

Blood?

When I looked down and saw crimson everywhere, I couldn't believe my eyes. I knew I needed help. The doctors on call at Roswell did, too. When Kenya and I arrived, it was a medical emergency. When the attending physician saw my heart rate and blood pressure, he said, "That can't be right."

He repeated the process. Again, he took my vitals—my body temperature, pulse, breathing rate, and blood pressure—and said, "I'll be right back." I couldn't breathe. My oxygen levels were dropping. My pulse and blood pressure were skyrocketing. Just then, nurses started showing up. The doctor walked into his small office.

Through blurry vision, I could see him pacing the floor, yapping away on the phone. My eyelids were involuntarily opening and closing, making my spying efforts difficult. I could hear him faintly speaking, but the words were hard to make out. I didn't know what the terminology he was using meant anyway.

But I gathered from his tone, body language, and overall panicked reaction, that patient Hobbs wasn't in good shape.

I WANTED TO GO HOME

They sent Kenya out and began their rectal examination. Let's just say, *ouch*, and leave it at that. I was wheeled into different rooms, laid under various machines and scanned multiple times. I was told again that my internal organs had seized up. Ken wasn't around this time. So they found their best chemotherapy nurse in the hospital to get my IV in. She was excellent, thank God.

Seeing her made me think about the words of my surgeon. He had me wondering, *Will I be needing chemo for colon cancer soon?* No, I wouldn't. That surgeon was wrong. He had to eat those words. "I know what I saw on your film," he said. "But it's not what I thought. There's nothing there but healthy tissue."

No cancer. No tumor. No polyps.

That good news came later. For now, I had to deal with this latest flare-up. I was dizzy, hurting and wishing for anything to knock me unconscious. A drug. A brick. A whack on the head. I really didn't care at that point. I just wanted a break from reality. For a while, I thought I might pass away before the team could finish their tests. It had gotten so bad, that idea was totally okay with me.

Going home—not my home on the outskirts of Buffalo, but in the heavenly realm—seemed like a pretty attractive proposition.

Being in a constant pain, the kind so excruciating I didn't know how to explain it verbally, was a lot. It wore me down. I had never been that low before. Chronic pain will try your will, test your strength and steal your fight like few other things can.

Though God was indeed holding me, I often could not feel His mighty and outstretched arms. I'd lay awake at night weeping and hoping death, which passed over the homes of the Israelites and spared their firstborn in Exodus 12, would knock on my door. I wished it would sweep me away in the night so I could wake up in paradise with no more pain.

I wanted to go home.

Home to be with the Lord.

I had gotten so morose about my predicament that I only found comfort in 2 Corinthians 5:8 NIV, which says, "We are confident, I say, and would prefer to be away from the body and at home with the Lord."

Transitioning to Heaven consumed me. I felt so defeated in this life, I thought my total healing would come through death. But it wasn't my time. God didn't let my conditions take me out. Rather, He took me through.

He got down in the valley of the shadow of death with me. And suddenly, the famous "Footprints in the Sand" poem became real. When I was suffering, He swept me up in His arms and carried me. After what I went through, Deuteronomy 1:31 ESV has especially profound meaning and symbolism for me when it says, "…the Lord your God carried you, as a man carries his son, all the way that you went until you came to this place."

DID HE REMEMBER ME?

The fact that He carried me doesn't mean I felt carried or supported at all times. I had moments when it felt like He dropped me hard. I know that was a mere feeling. While I was in the thick of it, however, time after time, I wondered, does He remember me?

Like Hannah in 1 Samuel 1:10, I released anguished, bitter cries. The agonizing, vicious spasms gripping every muscle in my body left me curled up like a fetus. Between moans, I uttered the same prayer the barren wife of Elkanah prayed in verse 11: "Look on your servant's misery and remember me."

Did He remember me?

As King Hezekiah did when he became mortally ill in Isaiah 38:2, I turned my face to the wall and made a petition. In verse 3 NIV, he said, "Remember, Lord, how I have walked before you faithfully and with wholehearted devotion and have done what is good in your eyes." For a time, it seemed the tears I shed were for naught. Nothing was changing, except for the worst. I questioned whether or not God saw my suffering. Have you ever felt that way, too?

Have you been in a place where you couldn't see God's plan and didn't understand why He allowed such torture day in, and day out? Maybe you're there now, in a rock-bottom state. It's rough, I know. You feel defeated. I did, too. But defeat wasn't my state of being.

I was the victor, even on my sick bed; yes, I was a victorious believer when it looked like I would never be delivered. I could not see how He would turn my sorrow into joy, my mourning into morning, and my test into a testimony.

But thank God almighty, He remembered me, just as He remembers you.

When you're sick, He remembers you. When your family is falling apart, He remembers you. When you're battling mental health and emotional issues, He remembers you. When the world forsakes you and those you love seem to have forgotten you, He remembers you.

HE WAS MAKING ME AN EFFECTIVE WITNESS

I now know my pain was purposeful. The humiliation had to precede the elevation.

The walk through the valley was important, so I could bring you with me to the depths of sorrow, as well as to the heights of joy. The pain was necessary for me, so that, through my life, you could see how God will use *your* present hurt for your future ministry.

He masterfully takes the loneliest, scariest, roughest, lowest places you've ever been and repurposes them as springboards into destiny.

Through my issues, He was making me an effective witness; an eyewitness; a firsthand witness; a tried-Him-and-I-know-Him-for-myself witness; an unshakeable witness; a you-can't-make-me-doubt-Him-I-know-too-much-about-Him witness; a you-can't-tell-it-like-I-can kind of witness.

His Word is not a fairytale. Jesus is alive. He saves. He delivers. He restores. He heals. Doctors didn't cure me, natural remedies didn't help me, surgery didn't spare me, and procedures didn't fix me.

It was the Lord *alone*.

Were it not for Him, where would I be?

As my pain began to crescendo, eventually reaching a level I could no longer stand, God said, *Enough!*

He considered me. He knew I had reached my maximum threshold. I couldn't take it another day. He remembered me and commanded affliction to release me, and it obeyed as quickly as the winds and waves calmed down at the word of Jesus in Mark 4:39.

When the fullness of time had come, the pain ceased. My system regulated. My symptoms disappeared.

God did it, just like that, and I will tell my testimony everywhere I go, to anyone that will listen. I will remind anyone suffering silently, crying frantically, hurting constantly, praying daily, believing consistently, but still being attacked viciously, that God remembers you.

You are not defeated. You are not invisible. You are not forsaken. You are already victorious. Your moment of triumph may take longer to get here than you want it to, just as mine did, but it will come.

BATTLING THE SPIRIT OF FEAR

Back at Roswell, prior to admitting me, the team agreed, "We've got to regulate her vitals." Though they were in agreement over what needed to be done for me, they didn't have an agreed upon method by which to accomplish that.

My vitals were feisty, stubborn and wholly uncooperative. They didn't want to be regulated. My system was screaming, trying to inform doctors that something was wrong. Those screams, which translated into pain, troubling blood pressure and heartrate spikes, were not going to stop until the underlying conditions were addressed.

But without sufficient knowledge of what the underlying conditions were, my case was hopeless. Before I knew it, I was being pumped full of who knows what. This would at least get the symptoms under control until their root causes could be found. One thing led to another, and Roswell soon became my temporary home. I had been physically body-slammed and defeated by unnamed, unregulated, unstoppable tormenters.

When I was cleared to go, I had a mixture of joyfulness and fearfulness, because, what landed me in the hospital was a ruthless, mysterious and threating combo. Who was to say those events wouldn't reoccur? When I was wheeled out of Roswell following my admittance, Kenya helped me into our vehicle.

On the way home, he kept asking, "Are you okay?"

"I'm fine," I told him, gripping his hand. What I *didn't* say was, I was battling the spirit of fear. I was petrified. When we arrived at the house, he tucked me in bed.

"The doctor said you need to eat something," he told me, as he administered my usual drug cocktail, along with a few new prescriptions. Consuming food was the last thing I wanted to do.

Not only was I not hungry, but I wasn't interested in putting anything on my stomach that might get trapped in my intestines. No thank you. Furthermore, swallowing was uncomfortable and nausea made food repulsive.

But Kenya wasn't taking no for an answer. He went to the kitchen and put 15 grapes in a Ziploc sandwich bag. When all else failed, that, or applesauce filled with Moringa, was the go-to meal.

Reluctantly, I bit into one of the sweet pieces of fruit, chewed it and managed to get it down my throat. One was all I could manage.

Kenya snuggled with me as I tried to drop off to sleep, but couldn't. I was fidgeting and ill at ease. Every time my heart beat more rapidly than usual, I was edgy and disquieted. "I'm scared," I finally admitted to Kenya. "What if the same thing that happened before happens again?"

"Don't think like that," he told me. "It's not going to happen again. You're going to be fine."

He always seemed to have the right answers. I scooted closer and latched onto his arm like a clingy cat. The warmth of his embrace offered a sense of physical security when nothing else was stable. He was a natural safe haven, while God was my spiritual refuge. I had to keep reminding myself moment by moment that, according to Romans 8:37, in all these things—even this thing known as failing health—I am more than a conqueror through Christ.

JESUS IS A BALM

God let me suffer for a season and stare defeat in the face so Christ, the undefeated One, could prove His supremacy, sovereignty and all-sufficiency through each trial.

Further, God let it happen knowing full well that, when He brought me out suddenly, this sold-out-for-Jesus girl would shout from the rooftop, *God did it!*

He knew I would barricade myself in a quiet room and write a book about the miracle by lamplight. I would willingly board flights around the world, tired and all, to tell everyone I could reach that Jesus is the true "Balm in Gilead" mentioned in Jeremiah 8.

In verse 20 of that chapter, the prophet Jeremiah said, "The harvest is past, the summer has ended, and we are not saved."

The season to be fruitful had come and gone, and yet, Judah saw no deliverance, no abundance, no prosperity, nothing but desolation, defeat, and sorrow. That verse sounds a little something like me prior to receiving healing.

In verse 22, Jeremiah cried out, "Is there no balm in Gilead? Is there no physician there? Why then is there no healing for the wound of my people?" He wanted to know, where was Judah's healing? Where was their restoration? Where was their relief? Where was their balm?

In the Old Testament, historians say, aromatic gum, also known as a spice used for healing, was very common. There was a bush notorious for producing the resin needed to make a special balm. This bush grew so plentifully in the land of Gilead that, in ancient times, the balm became known as the balm of Gilead.

For us, Jesus Christ is the Balm in Gilead.

He, unlike the natural, medicinal, ancient aromatic balm that came from plants, is unlimited. He heals *all* wounds—physical, emotional and psychological. Christ is not confined to the physical territory of Gilead, notorious for its spices and ointments, east of the Jordan River. The Balm in Gilead I know is far more effective than the top-quality ointment with soothing properties.

One drop of His blood is good enough to wash away sins, redeem fallen mankind back to God, wipe out whatever ails us, and secure eternal life for all who place their hope and trust in Him.

I got to know the Balm better in sickness, which makes me thankful for the affliction, hard as it was. I didn't like what I was subjected to. And no, God did not pad the bottom of my pit.

DOWN I WENT

He didn't give me a pillow to lie down on to soften the hardness of the rock and a hard place I was stuck between. He allowed me to feel the hurt—all of it.

He let me experience a sense of defeat.

I didn't get to avoid that sinkhole of melancholy and despondency. In my woeful state He wanted me to realize that man's balm could temporarily ease my dis-ease, but only the real Balm of Gilead could permanently cure me.

From deep in the doldrums, I cried, and He dried my eyes. When I tossed and turned, soaking the bed sheets with sweat and tears, He serenaded me with songs of Zion.

When I didn't understand why He didn't alleviate my pain, He calmed my spirit and strengthened me. When I called out His name in my distress, He did not make the treacherous, vindictive, merciless enemies that ripped me from limb to limb, stop, but He did not let them defeat me.

Stormy rains had turned my life's green grass into a muddy quagmire into which I sank.

Down I went, thinking I would never rise again. Through that, God revealed what true joy is. It is not the absence of pain, but the presence of God. He showed me what true victory is. It is not the absence of feelings of defeat, but the presence of God who is greater than those feelings.

God made sure I knew that His favor didn't mean I could avoid the deepest levels of affliction. In the Kingdom, it doesn't work like that. God is not the guarantor of a trouble-free life; He is a refuge in the time of trouble. He is not the promiser of a storm-free existence; He is shelter from the rain. He does not guarantee prevention of ailments and discomfort; but He is the Balm and deliverer.

FLAT-OUT LIED

I now understand that when oppositional forces threaten me, they will not defeat me, for the Lord is with me. Insurmountable odds create the right conditions for our undefeatable God to step in and do what He does best: work a miracle.

Satan has flat-out lied to you by telling you you're defeated.

He told me that fib, too. He crafted a fictitious story that set him up as the strong villain and made me out to be the weak victim. But our myth-busting God dispelled that erroneous tale. When the fullness of time had come, the Omniscient One flexed His power and exposed Satan for the liar he is.

You are a winner. You can't lose. Christ, the undefeated champion, has overcome. Whatever phase of the journey you're now in, you know how the story ends.

"But thanks be to God! He gives us the victory through our Lord Jesus Christ" (1 Corinthians 15:57 NIV).

A prayer for you: God, what this person is now going through makes it look like, in some areas, they are defeated. But You have already declared them victorious, despite the odds against them. In their darkest moments, when the silence and darkness envelope them, when a stormy sea of problems engulfs them, when the feeling that You are far away overwhelms them, pierce the darkness. Calm the raging seas. Hold them. Let them know that You are there and this is not the end.

I thank You that they are just days away from reaping their harvest of blessings and breakthrough. No weapon will prosper against them. They will walk through this valley and emerge as the victorious believer You have declared them to be; and it is not by might, nor by power, but by Your spirit, according to Zechariah 4:6.

For this I thank You and give you praise!

In Jesus' name, Amen.

PHASE SIX

CONFLICTED

A carnal mind cannot receive the wonderfulness of all God has in store.

I wish I could describe the phase I went through right before my healing as one that was anticipatory, confident and faith-filled. If I told you that, it would sound good, but it wouldn't be the authentic truth.

And by now, if you have read every page leading up to this one, you already know, I don't filter out what is true in favor of what is most palatable, pleasant or proper. I am not about to try to make myself look or sound better at the expense of honesty.

MY HYPOTHESIS

I had a conflict going on inside me, an internal war. As I walked through the meandering valley of sickness, part of me believed wholeheartedly that God, my healer, was going to work a supernatural miracle in my body. The other part of me expected my progress and recovery to be natural, and gradual.

I had a hypothesis.

It was this: the manmade balm we discussed in the previous chapter, and the Balm of Gilead, would tag-team my affliction and get me right once again.

That sounded theoretically plausible to me.

But here's the problem: what God wanted to do was *implausible*. So, yeah, there's that. He had to inform me that my speculative theory was wrong. He disproved my little uneducated thesis in a dream.

In my sleep, God appeared to me. He was very tall and I could not see His face, but I knew it was Him. He held my hand as we slowly walked and talked. During our one-on-one exchange, He told me He was going to heal me.

I responded by telling God I believed He would do it, but it would be part practical, part miraculous.

The God of the universe shot my idea down like a marksman aiming at soda cans during target practice. I watched it fall to the ground and fizzle. The Lord said, no, my healing would be "all miraculous."

Again, I protested as if Dianna Hobbs, a mere mortal, knew better than the One who had formed and fashioned me in my mother's womb.

"No, it will be part practical, part miraculous," I shot back.

God, who was patient and loving, but firm, in this dream I had just weeks before my instantaneous healing, told me the third time, "It will be all miraculous."

Seeing that He was unflinching, I finally conceded, "Okay, well, if you say it's going to be all miraculous, I believe you. It'll be all miraculous."

Even as I was uttering those words to God in my sleep, my feelings opposed what I verbalized. In this prophetic dream, my decision to give up my *part practical, part miraculous* position wasn't rooted in faith, per se. It was more so a recognition that I can't argue with God. If He said it, whether or not my thoughts and emotions agreed, I had to surrender my position and accept His will. What He was proposing was too farfetched and much too wonderful to grasp with my carnal, natural, human way of thinking.

As far out and far off as a miracle seemed to be, I still woke up the next day with excitement coursing through my veins. I also had lots of confusion clouding my brain.

All miraculous? I thought. *How is that going to happen?*

I didn't have an answer, of course. God didn't tell me the how, when, or where. Only the what. So I held the promise in my heart, even with all those questions swirling around in my head.

IT HAD BEEN A LONG TIME COMING

In part, my struggle to believe for a suddenly-shift in my circumstances was so hard because change had been a long time coming. My battle with an eye disease that God subsequently healed me from was the beginning of my journey. The Glaucoma diagnosis was in early 2015. Two years later, I was still in the throes of this battle with sickness. I had been praying for months and months with no change.

I know there are others that waited a *very* long time—far longer than I did—for healing. Some went decades. Others are still in the wait. By comparison, my process, which took a couple years in total, was fairly short. Also, the most intense pain, the kind that made it impossible for me to function, showed up about six months before my healing.

So I know that, comparatively speaking, I am blessed that it wasn't worse for me.

And yet, when pain is aggressive, it can make a day feel like a thousand years. As the saying goes, "Time flies when you're having fun." I'd like to add to that: it crawls when you're not. The waiting period felt like an eternity.

In 2016, when the forces of darkness ramped up the attack, the intensity caught me off guard. I had been keeping the situation under wraps, still blogging, vlogging, podcasting, encouraging others, and living life. All that was getting ready to come to a screeching halt.

I'd underestimated my enemy and overestimated my natural ability to fight at first. That's a mistake we often make. We bring a knife to a gunfight. We show up with a carnal mindset, unaware that we are embroiled in a spiritual battle royal.

I HAD NEVER FELT ANYTHING LIKE THAT BEFORE

The first time I saw a huge bruise on one of my calves, I didn't view it as a sign of trouble. I was actually dismissive. I reasoned that the discolored tender spot resulted from my own clumsiness.

I must have hit my leg while working out without noticing, I thought. I was right that I had been hit, but the blow was not external. There was something devastating happening internally, and the contusion was only the earliest visible symptom.

Though I had been battling chronic fatigue for months, suffering with digestive issues, needing midday naps, and frequently contracting what I assumed were viruses, I didn't jump to conclusions. I had seen my primary physician, who recommended consuming more water, fruits, vegetables, and reducing stress levels. I obeyed.

As days passed, I reckoned my ailments would pass also. That way of thinking changed on September 23, 2016. It was our oldest son Kedar's 13th birthday. I was sitting at the table during his at-home party when a burning and stabbing pain shot through both arms. Heat and sharp spasms made it feel as if voltage wires had been clamped to my blood vessels.

What in the world were these piercing, extreme sensations shooting through me?

I had never felt anything like that before and hoped I never would again.

That hope would be repeatedly dashed in the coming days, weeks and months.

I quickly surveyed the laughter-filled room to ensure our happy-go-lucky troops didn't suspect I was in a bad way that Saturday night. I didn't want to ruin the festive mood where Kyla, Kaiah and Kaleb were having loads of fun with their brother. I prayed none of them noticed me grimacing. Unable to keep up the fakery another second, I bolted up the steps. Tears were welling up, threatening to out me.

Thankfully, I escaped our small dining area just off the kitchen before waterworks escaped my eyes. I took refuge in my bedroom. Shortly thereafter, Kenya, who suspected something wasn't right, emerged.

"What's wrong?" he queried.

I tried explaining, but words failed me. That piercingly sad look in his eyes meant he was troubled and perplexed. I couldn't find anything in my vocabulary to sufficiently express what I felt.

All that came out is, "Something is wrong. Something is really wrong."

Then came another strike. "My neck!" I shouted, grabbing at it and running into our master bathroom to gaze at it in the mirror. I'm not sure what I was looking for exactly, but I didn't expect what I saw. My right external jugular vein was bulging, tightening like a rubber band that had been stretched too far.

The throbbing and discomfort was so great I grew dizzy. Just before keeling over, Kenya caught me.

"I think you might have to go to the ER," he said. "This isn't normal."

Feeling faint, winded and foggy-headed, I still mustered the strength to protest. "I can't do that," I responded, shaking my head, unwilling to seek medical treatment right then. I didn't want to ruin the celebratory atmosphere of Kedar's special day. I had been rushed to the hospital on our daughter's birthday once before with a broken arm. I wasn't trying to make ER visits regular birthday traditions.

OUT-OF-BODY EXPERIENCE

In 2011, in celebration of Kyla's birthday, on February 4th, we held a party at a local skating rink. I fell while skating and sustained a distal radius fracture, or more simply, a broken wrist. The bone completely snapped in half and damaged my joints and cartilage.

Initially, I thought I'd only be in a cast for a couple of months, but the damage from the fall I tried to break with my outstretched arm and open hand, required surgery. I had to have a metal plate and screws permanently inserted to fuse the bone back together.

My surgeon assured me the healing process would take a few weeks. But things went very wrong. After what should have been a straightforward and uncomplicated surgical procedure, I went into cardiac arrest and had a near-death experience.

The details I'm sharing with you here are a mix of what I remember and the blanks filled in for me by the medical staff.

I woke up after surgery, crying out in pain. It felt like someone had lit a match, setting my arm on fire, while simultaneously banging it with a hammer. Although I could barely see anything, I recall hearing myself screaming, as well as a nurse saying, "Calm down. You're going into shock. I need you to calm down and breathe!"

I tried to breathe. I truly did my best.

But I felt breath leaving my body.

"God, please don't let me die," I begged.

I knew something was amiss. I could sense it. Suddenly, I was having an out-of-body experience. I was carried away to this gorgeously lush green pasture. The sky was bluer than anything I'd ever witnessed.

There was a beautiful tree in full bloom. The grass was filled with small daisies. The sun was brighter than bright. I felt at peace. I was no longer in any pain. I was wearing a flowing white night gown and was barefoot. I was laughing, happy and free.

All of a sudden, an internal alarm went off. It warned me that, despite how serene the atmosphere in this middle-of-nowhere field was, it was *not* where I was supposed to be. I saw the faces of our four children flash before me.

It looked like someone had taken a stack of Polaroid photos, spread them out, suspended them in mid-air, and flipped them in rapid succession. Snapshots of every phase of the kids' lives, from infancy to their current age, popped up one after another at the speed of lightning.

My tranquility was interrupted by inner-panic. I suddenly didn't like this utopia.

CODE BLUE!

How had I gotten there? Why did it feel like my life was ending? I had reached an impasse of sorts. There seemed to be no way out of this place. But I couldn't leave Kyla, Kaiah, Kedar and Kaleb behind. My babies needed their mom.

As my body, currently in shock, lay deathly still, I had this overwhelming urge to fight to stay. I couldn't move any body parts or open my eyes, but my sense of hearing was keen. My heart rate shot up and kept climbing. We had a real issue. I was going through some serious changes.

I heard myself take three shallow breaths. *Who's turning off the oxygen valve?* I wondered. I had less and less air to breathe. Interestingly, the sensation of not being able to inhale wasn't uncomfortable. I didn't feel like I was suffocating.

I simply was losing air. A frantic female voice shouted out, "We've got a Code Blue!"

I thought, *Code Blue? I know they can't be talking about me.*

But, they were, in fact, talking about me. Code Blue is called out in a hospital when a patient is in cardiopulmonary arrest. The "code team" rushes to the area and starts resuscitative efforts. I've seen this scenario play out on television shows and in movies, but this was real life. It was *my* life. I was in cardiac arrest. I could hear the commotion but was paralyzed.

It's the weirdest feeling to have an active mind, but an inactive body. *Hey! I can hear you over here,* I was trying to say. Just then, God and I started up an internal dialogue. Physically, I was completely immobile, but I was fully engaged mentally, emotionally and spiritually.

PRAYER BROUGHT ME BACK

I prayed—more like groveled.

"Please don't take me away from my children," I silently uttered my plea. And that's when I heard the strong voice of God say, "You've got people praying for you."

I will never forget those words. I never again viewed intercessory prayer the same after hearing them come from my Heavenly Father's mouth. After He spoke that, it was lights out. Everything went black. All my senses shut down.

Next thing I remember is blinking and seeing a blurry face coming into focus. A pair of distraught eyes were looking back at me. They belonged to a nurse who was tightly gripping my right hand. I fought to maintain consciousness as she begged me to breathe and stay awake. But my eyes and my body felt heavy. I drifted in and out.

I later learned that, for five minutes, the medical team couldn't get me back. If it had not been for the grace of God, I would not be here today.

Prayer brought me back.

The intercessory prayers of the righteous that the Bible characterizes as "powerful and effective" in James 5:16 NIV, took effect.

After regaining a sense of who I was and where I was, I saw that tubes and wires were hanging from every place. I was confused and bewildered. *Who put all this stuff all over me?* I wondered. *How did it happen without my knowledge? What was going on?*

"You gave us quite the scare," the nurse told me. "You should have seen all the doctors surrounding your bed!"

What she didn't know is that it was not the doctors, but the angels of the Lord surrounding my bed. God resuscitated me and gave me more time. It was the power of prayer that raised me up.

Once I was released and sent home, my recovery was brutal. It took months instead of weeks. Aside from the physical injury, the side effects of being without oxygen to my brain for an extended period, were severe.

I had memory loss, heart trouble, mobility issues and digestive problems. My body wasn't working. Doctors didn't know how to help me. What should have been an easy recovery from a fracture, turned into sheer physical, emotional and psychological chaos.

After surviving that, I assumed it would be the toughest physical storm I'd ever have to weather. But five years later, a new, fiercer battle presented itself, and upped the ante. With my wrist-breaking saga in rearview, I assumed my recovery from my autoimmune diseases would mimic that process.

There were certain portions of my 2011 struggle that mirrored my autoimmunity crisis: I had to take medicine and battle chronic pain for months, I was bedridden for a time, and I lost an extreme amount of weight. Then, slowly but surely, God gave me some relief.

Although the nerve, joint and tendon damage done to my left hand during my fall still remains, I am able to function. It took over a year after I injured the limb to be able to grab things again. I regained about 80 percent limb functionality and some of my memory.

But still, if I try to isolate just the pointer, middle and ring fingers on my left hand, I cannot straighten them. They appear crooked and malformed. Surgeons want to operate again; I told them no. There are also some people and things I no longer remember following my post-surgical complications. I never regained certain memories I lost.

I STRUGGLED TO BELIEVE

You see, *those* are the details stored in my mental library. I didn't realize it at first, but I had let them shape how I viewed healing.

The reason why I expected a part practical, part miraculous process, is because that's what happened before. The miraculous part of what occurred in 2011 is that God brought me back from death's door. The practical part is, the healing and recovery took lots of prayer and time, and physical therapy.

By allowing that 2011 experience to influence my thinking so much, I struggled to believe for the new thing He wanted to do.

My previous ordeal taught me to be realistic and measured in my expectations. It told me that my dilemma will likely cause permanent damage and result in lifelong limitations. My fingers were my evidence. My memory loss was proof.

But God did not ask me to go into my mental library to search out historical data by which to classify and qualify what He was about to do, did He? It was my misguided attempt to anticipate God's methods that led to me boxing Him in.

Little did I know, He had an unprecedented miracle in store for me. My notion that my history determined my destiny was wrong.

God was not and is not limited by what I have witnessed in previous circumstances. That was then; this is now. He was telling me, "For I am about to do something new. See, I have already begun! Do you not see it?" (Isaiah 43:19 NLT)

Don't make the mistake I made. Don't ever think that because you have never seen it, God won't ever do it. Also, don't get stuck in yesterday. God is always up to something fresh, different and brand new.

We can never predict how He will move. There are unexpected breakthroughs with your name on them. There are miracles that He will perform for you. There are cycles He is going to break in your life. Just because it didn't happen for you last time, doesn't indicate that it won't happen next time. My life is a witness.

You have no reference point for the amazing blessings that are on the way to you. "But as Scripture says: 'No eye has seen, no ear has heard, and no mind has imagined the things that God has prepared for those who love him'" (1 Corinthians 2:9 GWT).

HOW HAD IT COME TO THIS?

I retraced my steps by looking back over the past several months. How had it come to this? How did I get to the place where I needed an emergency prayer service?

I stared at a red chair up against one of our bedroom walls. It was the one I'd sat down in the first night neuropathic pain shot through my arms on Kedar's birthday. That had been six months ago. I had not imagined a reality so grim awaited me in the not-so-distant future.

I was sucked into a time warp. My mind carried me back to Kedar's birthday all over again. I had laid on Kenya's shoulder weeping. He'd knelt in front of the red chair and stroked my back.

"You're going to be okay, honey," he assured me—a line he had said hundreds of times since, and was still saying. Through the most harrowing health battle of our lives, sometimes with teary eyes, and a shaky voice, Kenya never stopped encouraging me.

I didn't know at the time how torn up inside he was until he later told me. He was being strong for me and the kids. My best friend, who I would marry all over again, was just as unwavering in faith toward the end as he was in the beginning.

But he'll readily admit, neither he nor I knew September 2016 was a negative turning point in our lives. After Kenya prayed for me upstairs in our bedroom, away from the children that were downstairs playing, I lifted my head and wiped my eyes. I was relieved that the symptoms had subsided, but terror-stricken at the thought of the pain coming back.

Boy, if I had only known. I'm glad I didn't. I'd crossed a new threshold. I was at the point of no return. There was still some muscle tightness after Kenya interceded that fall evening. But the electric-shock-like pain ceased for a time. After the party was over, I had one more thing to do before turning in.

I broke my silence for the first time. The cover-up phase we discussed in a previous chapter ended at that moment. I called my mother around bedtime.

Let me take you inside that call.

I had a simple plan: calmly tell her I wasn't feeling well and request prayer. Easy-peasy. I assumed I could keep the full magnitude of my dilemma under wraps and avoid tipping her off if I played it cool.

Where did I get that idea? I should have known better.

I LOST IT

A mother knows her child, which is why my first inclination was to saying nothing. But this was a 9-1-1 emergency. I had to beef up the spiritual counterattack on this evil foe. But there was no way to coolly and collectedly solicit intercessory prayers.

This is owed to the fact that my mother, the sweetest woman on this side of heaven, has an uncanny knack for unveiling secrets.

Her hugs are warmer than quilts, comforters and fleece blankets combined. Howbeit, Mother Annie Brinson doesn't have to physically touch anyone to get them to open up.

Her genuine concern and sympathetic tone consistently melt away tough exteriors. Whether I wanted it to happen or not, the truth, like candle wax held to a flame, came dripping off my tongue.

"I'm in so much pain and I don't know what's wrong!" I bawled and wailed.

I lost it.

I turned into an undignified, hysterical, emotional train wreck, whose pleas for intercession were almost unintelligible. It was the full-on ugly cry, the kind of sobbing that makes it hard to understand what in the world a person is saying. I was heaving like I'd just gotten one of Daddy's infamous whippings I dreaded as a child.

You would have thought someone pulled out the leather belt and went to town on my hind parts.

Even though Mom couldn't make out every word, she knew I was in distress. I sat in bed clutching the receiver. My forehead rested in my clammy right palm and a lake of tears spilled onto my t-shirt.

I detailed the all-over-my-body aching and bruising, night sweats, and pain-induced insomnia I was suffering with daily.

"Please pray for me," I desperately begged. "I don't know what's happening and I'm tired."

I AM INTENSELY PRIVATE

I needed that belly-shaking, eyes-will-be-puffy-in-the-morning, from-the-depths-of-my-soul, cleansing cry. It had been welling up from within and finally came bursting forth in the form of a confession.

When the prayer circle grew as a result of that impromptu tearful confessional, it made me uncomfortable. I was conflicted about opening up. When it comes to personal things, I am intensely private. But nothing gets you to drop your guard like a painful attack of the enemy.

Before the tsunami of emotions rushed the shores of my pride, knocking down the walls I'd built up and forcing my safely secured secrets out into the open, I was a different woman. I didn't let anyone in. I carried weight on my shoulders. I talked myself out of asking for help, no matter how much I needed it.

I don't like to bother anyone. I don't wish to impose. I prefer independence to co-dependence. I want to be an asset, not a liability; a blessing, not a burden. But God used my ordeal to open me up and teach me that, sometimes, co-dependency is good.

No woman or man is an island unto themselves. Everybody needs somebody.

GOD WAS TAKING ME HIGHER

As conflicted as I felt about sharing my battle then, I understand now how important it was. The Lord was using my situation to publicly glorify Himself. He was not going to waste my pain.

Out of it, He was birthing purpose. I needed to stop being carnal and get out of my flesh. When the diseases presented themselves, Satan used them to come against my faith and make me give up hope.

God used these problems another way: to reveal who He is and who I am in Him. He was taking me higher.

I had reached a plateau in my journey of faith, and God was taking me to a greater level; the only way to get me there was to allow me to be tried in the fire. He permitted me to engage in a literal fight for my life.

He knew the epic duel would transform me into a bold, Kingdom warrior, unafraid to believe Him for the impossible things that no words can explain.

I now walk in a new level of faith. There's nothing like *seeing firsthand* what God can do.

A little earlier, I mentioned Hezekiah, the righteous king of Judah who became deathly ill in Isaiah 38. He sought God tearfully after being told he would die. In response to Hezekiah's anguished plea, something shifted.

The Lord sent a word to the king through the Prophet Isaiah. He said, "I have heard your prayer and seen your tears; I will add fifteen years to your life."

But God didn't stop there. There was more good news. He also told Hezekiah, in reference to his formidable and intimidating opponent, Sennacherib, King of Assyria, "I will deliver you and this city from the hand of the king of Assyria. I will defend this city."

And the Lord made good on both promises. Not only did He heal Hezekiah, but the Lord defeated the Assyrians, too. God turned everything around, which shows us that when things look their worst, He is able to work them out for the best. One minute, the king was facing death.

The next, after God sent a word, he got his health and his life back. There was a suddenly-shift in Hezekiah's situation. And mine.

Perhaps your circumstances look horrible. All you're hearing is bad news. Everything around you appears to be falling apart and you're thinking, Dianna, I don't see any end to the negative cycle of problems, disappointments and challenges.

I've been where you are. But God is speaking the words He said to Hezekiah to you today: "I have heard your prayer and seen your tears." Know that He is going to shift things in your favor.

So, save yourself the stress and worry. Take it from me; it's not necessary. I have, in the past, exhausted myself with worry. It changes nothing. Instead of focusing on the formidableness of your opponent, shift your attention to the greatness of your God. Let Him take your faith to another level.

FOCUS YOUR EYES ON THE SAVIOR

Quit looking at your situation; whenever I did that, my stomach knotted and my faith flip-flopped. Fearing your opponent instead having faith in the One who can defeat that opponent, will leave you anxiety-ridden, conflicted, and tense.

Focus your eyes on the Savior and place your confidence in His power over your problems. Then that conflict will give way to peace. Then that worry will give way to faith.

Then you will boldly declare the words found in Romans 8:31 NIV, which says, "What, then, shall we say in response to these things? If God is for us, who can be against us?"

> *A prayer for you: God, the person reading right now wasn't expecting a blow like this; life wasn't supposed to be this hard. These setbacks have presented numerous challenges. They thought the promises You made would have come to pass by now.*
>
> *The letdowns have been soul-crushing and have delivered firm blows to their faith. They want to believe You, but their emotions are embattled and their feelings are conflicted.*
>
> *But thank You for reigniting both their faith and their fight. In weak moments, remind them that, according to 2 Corinthians 10:4, the weapons we fight with are not the*

carnal weapons of the world, but they are mighty through You, and have divine power to demolish strongholds.

I touch and agree with them by faith. We proclaim, together, that You are picking up the pieces of their lives, collecting all the ashes, and turning them into something beautiful for Your glory.

In Jesus' name, we give You thanks, Amen.

PHASE SEVEN

HEALED
And just like that, God did it.

Before my miracle happened, I had a few clues about what God was up to. The "all miraculous" dream tipped me off, but it was baffling at best.

Though I know how to believe God for miraculous things, somewhere along the way, I must admit, I had stopped regularly exercising my faith muscles. I had slipped into a zone of complacency. But my sickness forced me to put a demand on the faith lying dormant.

God knew what was in me and was aware that a fiery trial would bring it out of me.

STEP-BY-STEP

At first, I was out of practice in the believe-big department. I needed some oiling. I was a bit rusty. I was something like a toddler just learning to use her legs: wobbly with the first few steps.

I felt unsure.

So God, who is gentle and patient, took me slowly. He began revealing more of His plan and His prowess by degrees. Little-by-little, step-by-step, He led me. He kept dropping breadcrumbs in the forest for me to follow that would ultimately lead me through the door to the healing He'd promised me.

God had been giving me amazing appetizers, whetting my appetite for the main course. He did it with Mr. Czarnecki, a man I have never met personally, who went out of his way to unlock the best treatment avenues for me. God did it again when He revealed to my dad that I was suffering with Fibromyalgia during his prayer time, before my rheumatologist knew.

My Heavenly Father flashed another entrée of divine favor before me when doctors stumbled across a tumor in the middle of a procedure. It had been hiding deep within my tissue. They thought the discovery was an accident. I knew better. That abnormal growth had been causing all kinds of pain and havoc. Surgeons assumed it was cancer, but God said, *no*. After surgery, I was told the good news: it was benign.

By the time the Lord revealed the same vision He gave me for the prayer service to Wynetta and moved on her heart to make it happen, the breadcrumbs got me even closer to my freedom from affliction. He had boosted my faith muscles quite a bit. My capacity to believe for greater kept growing with each supernatural manifestation.

I saw God's sovereign hand and presence all throughout my dilemma. There are just too many miracles to describe and contain them all in this one book. I could write volumes.

Now the moment had come to swallow the main course. No more appetizers. No more baby steps. No more gradual unveilings. It was time for the grand finale. I had to believe God for that sweeping, cure-all, skip-all-the-steps, and change-everything-in-an-instant type miracle that would stump and stupefy me. I had to get my expectations up for Him to do it.

EVERYTHING WAS A STRUGGLE

At this point, I was a shell of my former self, barely hanging on by a thread. My mom and sisters were pitching in where they could to help out at my house. On Thanksgiving, for instance, my sister Shavette, who is one of the most compassionate, selfless, giving people I know, made dinner for my family and hers. She's an amazing cook and a multi-faceted creative person.

She is closest to me in age and was always the caretaker of our family when we were growing up. Shavette was my first and only beautician. She beat up my bullies for me in school. She made all the decorations for my wedding. And she did all she could to cheer me up, support me and encourage me when I was sick.

Being cheerful was a struggle some days.

Everything was a struggle.

But one of my sisters could make me laugh and laugh, and laugh some more. I would giggle with abandon until I didn't feel the aches that had been plaguing me all day. She'd having me wiping away tears, not from sadness, but from silliness. My younger sister Alesha, a singer, playwright, and undercover comedian, would come by to see me.

When I was confined to my bed, she'd drop by with the same three things: a large order of McDonald's fries, a large sweet tea, and a ton of laughter. When nobody could get me to eat, Alesha would do her best to tempt my taste buds, and when I didn't have a whole lot to smile about, she worked extra hard to tickle my funny bone. She almost *always* succeeded, too. She remains one of the funniest people I know— just silly for no reason.

One evening, I had a dream about Alesha: I was in a hospital bed, hooked up to an IV. She had on a white coat and was the attending physician, but instead of putting medicine in my drip, she was shooting up my veins with laughter. I was in no pain; her treatment proved effective.

Proverbs 17:22 NIV is true: "A cheerful heart is good medicine, but a crushed spirit dries up the bones." In the final days leading up to my healing service, my spirit was crushed. I needed all the laughter, sunshine and pick-me-ups I could get.

My mom helped cook holiday feasts, too. She'd take over my kitchen and whip up some delectable dishes. I was sad I couldn't do it myself, but no less filled with thanksgiving that my family did all they could to help me maintain some semblance of normalcy in the Hobbs household. I'll never forget their labor of love.

NO MORE HOPE FOR ME

By this point, my diseases had progressed so much, I couldn't do anything. I never went outside unless I had a doctor's appointment or medical emergency requiring a hospital visit.

The more time passed, the more critical things got. My rapid decline accelerated even more. In March 2017, weeks before my healing, this is where it got the hardest.

My day of reckoning came when, in the natural, it appeared to be all over for me. There was no more hope for me.

"I'm sorry. There's nothing else we can do for you," my specialist told me. He was the last one that promised he could help after all the others threw their hands up. Of all people, not him. He couldn't be saying this to me! I was gobsmacked to hear those words. Quite honestly, they didn't really register in my brain.

I remember thinking, *is he giving up on me, just like that—really?*

That day in March, I was particularly discouraged because I was in so much pain. My body had deteriorated. My clothes were no longer fitting. I had lost most of the mobility in my legs. I couldn't digest food. My voice wasn't working. My digestive system had gone kaput. My fluid-filled joints were swollen. My blood pressure was at stroke levels. The pain was blinding.

"Can he do that?" I asked my husband, who was taken aback by the staggering news as well. "They can just give up on me like that? Is that legal?"

When I think about that day with a clear head, I think, *Did I really ask about the legality of the doctor's decision to stop treatment?* Desperation will make you question everything. But at the time, the aching was so severe, I felt it was nothing short of criminal to send me on my way with no solutions. I was informed that the best they could hope for was to keep me comfortable.

A wrecking ball had just plowed through the wall and crushed my spirit.

Life was over.

I was going to die.

I needed to find a way to say goodbye to my husband, children and loved ones. It was time to get my affairs in order, because I didn't have long; that's what Satan said. He wanted the doctor's negative report to erase my mind, so I'd forget God's promise that my healing would be "all miraculous."

It would have to be, because practically speaking, my four decades on earth would end shortly in fatality.

I WASN'T QUITE READY TO GO

Every drug they had failed. This elite specialist, who gave up that day, had previously been so confident in his methods, he promised to make me better within 24 hours.

He apparently had never seen a case like mine.

He said he didn't even know of anyone to refer me to. The doctor who was treating me before him suggested *this guy*—this guy who was now telling me I was beyond help.

When I got back home, I cried and cried. Previously, I wanted to die, or so I thought.

When actually faced with the real prospect of dying, I wasn't quite ready to go.

I thought about what I would be leaving behind. I felt like there was more Kingdom work for me to do. My heart shattered.

While defenseless and absolutely broken, my heartless chief adversary saw an opportunity to challenge the one last thing I had to hold onto: the promises of God.

Satan told me I had imagined that dream about my "all miraculous" healing. It was a figment of my imagination. A manifestation of my subconscious desires, not a message from God.

While he was steadily beating me down, Kenya was persistently building me up. My husband chiseled away at Satan's lies with a powerful weapon of war: God's word.

He shared scriptures. He reminded me of prophecies.

Kenya asked me, "Why would God have you rally all these intercessors to pray if He wasn't going to heal you?"

The "50 Women Praying" service was a couple weeks away now. The stage was set. The wheels were already in motion. And Heaven was on my side.

But I didn't feel like it.

A DEAD DOG

I could identify with Mephibosheth of the Bible when he referred to himself as a "dead dog." I know that's a pretty harsh description, but, with all he had been through, that's simply the way he felt.

At just five years old, his father and grandfather were both killed in war. After learning the awful news, the boy's terrified nurse took off running, and in her haste, she accidentally dropped him.

He fell so hard, he was left crippled. Unable to get around and enjoy life like his peers, Mephibosheth, the son of Jonathan, David's former best friend, and grandson of King Saul, felt dead and useless. But God was not through with him.

In 2 Samuel 9, *years* after the incident that disabled him for life, David, now king, remembered his promise to show loyalty and kindness to those in Saul's lineage. He sought out any living relatives, and upon finding Mephibosheth, David gave him the full inheritance of Saul and his family.

The harvest now belonged to him, and he would always be a guest at King David's table (verses 9-10).

When Mephibosheth was found, he was in a place called Lodebar. In Hebrew, it means "no pasture." There was no fruitfulness and it was a dry place; but God's favor changed all that. The Lord caused rivers of blessings to flow through Mephibosheth's desert dwelling, and at long last, he got his harvest.

I, too, was in Lodebar, a dry place with no pasture, feeling as useless as a dead dog, all the while believing God to reap a harvest. Life was one big paradox; I was confessing that I was healed by Jesus's stripes, as disease preyed upon me, and death stalked me. I proclaimed victory while I was engaged in an active war with the enemy, being pelted with bullets from all sides.

Things made no sense, kind of like an oxymoron, which is a phrase or figure of speech that's incongruent or contradictory. The very nature of the word perfectly captures its meaning. Oxymoron is derived from the Greek, 'oxy,' meaning sharp, and 'moron' signifying something 'dull'—two opposing meanings.

There are an abundance of examples of oxymoronic word combinations, such as: deafening silence, perfectly imperfect, jumbo shrimp, awfully good, definite maybe, bittersweet, and pretty ugly.

That last one just about sums up my situation. Things had gotten pretty ugly, but I was on the brink of experiencing something awfully good.

THE NIGHT OF MY HEALING

It was Sunday, March 26, 2017. The intercessors had gathered at the church, but I was still in the hotel room, trying to get it together. I remember calling my sister, Shavette, struggling to get words out between sobs. I don't even know how she made out what I was saying; between the hoarseness of my barely-there voice and the over-emotionalism that choked my every word, I must have sounded like a muddled mess.

"Vette, I don't feel like I can make it, I'm so sick. I can't get myself together," I said as my body quivered. If the slightest breeze had blown through the bathroom where I sat, I would have tipped over.

She told me, "You can do it, Dianna. I'm here waiting for you." Just as she had been the whole time, she was there for me that day, too.

And, oh, how I needed her.

That evening, for the first time, the children saw their mother break down. I couldn't stop the fountain of tears or stabilize my shaking body; I was out of sorts, out of strength and out of character. I'm usually able to pull it together, but Satan didn't want me to make it to the service that night, so he ramped up the attack.

"I don't think I can make it," I told Kenya, on the verge of giving up the fight. But I'll never forget the words he said to me through tears. We were both crying as a matter of fact.

"You are only moments away from your miracle," he told me with intensity, passion, faith and conviction. He was prophesying to me.

DRY BONES

I was weak, but through those eight prophetic words Kenya spoke into my life, God breathed on me in the same manner that He breathed on that valley of dry bones in Ezekiel 37.

In verse 6, He prophesied to those bones, saying, "I will put breath in you, and you will come to life. Then you will know that I am the Lord."

My dry bones were about to come to life, too; but before they did, I had to press my way to the church.

Thank God I made it!

When Kenya pulled up, Shavette was right there with a warm smile, telling me I could do this, and that so many people had come out just to pray for me. Minister Marquis Robertson was standing there as well, helping me when I nearly fell over.

I first met Marquis in May 2010 at a department store called Sears at the Galleria Mall, on the outskirts of Buffalo. I was a woman on a mission that day. I had to sing at a banquet with a mandatory dress code: a dressy hat. I didn't own one, so off to the mall I went.

When I asked the friendly employee, Marquis, if he could direct me to where the hats were, he kindly showed me the way with a bright smile.

Then this helpful stranger said something that took me by surprise: he told me how much he loved my blog, *Your Daily Cup of Inspiration*, and that he was a faithful reader. He also told me one of the hats I was considering buying looked a mess.

We laughed heartily; he told no lies about the hat.

We have remained connected ever since. I was so glad to see him the night of my prayer service, with the same friendly smile he greeted me with in 2010.

When I entered the sanctuary of Covenant of Grace, it felt like an out-of-body experience. More accurately, it seemed like I had a lead role in a sad drama that evoked tears, head shakes and sympathetic looks from audience members.

I have never liked being the center of attention, so the fact that one of the worst moments of my life was being put on display felt particularly torturous.

I wished my dry bones could carry me. I wanted to walk myself in. But here was no way I could do it.

HE TOOK ME TO THE KING

I wanted to be alone, anywhere other than this place where the hot gaze of hundreds of pairs of eyes were burning holes in my feeble back. Most of the attendees hadn't seen me in months, some in *years*; needless to say, this was not the reunion I wanted.

But the news of my malady spread like an infectious airborne virus. It moved through homes, churches, offices, virtual networks, across state lines and on different continents; it went around the world.

A stampede of believers stormed Heaven to pray for me; they carried me in their hearts as Kenya carried me in his arms. My tender and attentive spouse did whatever he had to do to get me to Jesus, knowing I was too feeble in body and mind to make it on my own.

I will never forget the security, strength and stability Kenya provided by scooping me up and allowing his legs to work for me, as my own body worked against me.

It reminds me of the beautiful story in Mark 2:1-12 where people banded together to help someone in need. A man was paralyzed and could not, on his own, get to Jesus. But four men, with hearts full of compassion, carried him on a mat to the house where the Savior was preaching.

Unfortunately, when they got there, Jesus was thronged by a crowd, leaving no way to reach the One who had power to heal the immobilized man. Refusing to be deterred, the Bible says they cut a hole in the roof and lowered the man's mat down through that manmade opening. They placed him right in front of Jesus, disrupting the Master's sermon.

Jesus, who was impressed with the four compassionate men's faith, healed the paralyzed man. Verse 12 (NLT) says, "And the man jumped up, grabbed his mat, and walked out through the stunned onlookers. They were all amazed and praised God, exclaiming, 'We've never seen anything like this before!'"

Those are the exact words so many of the attendees of my prayer service said: *we've never seen anything like this before.* It was a sight to behold, a humbling, mind-blowing sight. Just like the paralyzed man in Mark 2, my healing was possible because someone willingly carried me to the Master.

That someone was Kenya.

He took me to the King.

Before I ran out of the sanctuary leaping and dancing, I entered weeping and hurting. I remember burying my face in Kenya's neck, hoping to hide my tears. That didn't work, though, as each teardrop encased a silent scream and broadcast it to the room.

However, what immediately offered comfort was the song I heard playing as I entered; it was Richard Smallwood's "Healing," one of my favorite songs. My baby sister, Shawndeanna, had coordinated a praise dance to it at my request.

It says, "There is a Balm in Gilead to heal the soul." Jesus, the Balm, was about to do what He does best. In Mark 2, it was for the man on the mat; this time, He was doing it for me.

Shawndeanna not only lent her gifts to the service that night, but she had been praying and uplifting me behind the scenes throughout the process. She is responsible for the existence of a Facebook Live video that has been viewed thousands of times online.

I was at my parents' kitchen table the night after God healed me, discussing the amazingness of the miracle He performed. I was crying and praising God when Shawndeanna pulled out her phone and began streaming that conversation. She made it possible for others to be a part of the intimate, celebratory moment. I didn't know she was recording at first, but now I'm so glad she did. I have revisited that video many times and tearfully relived the moment.

In it, I tell a story about how, earlier that day, I was looking for something in my purse. When I reached down in my handbag, I felt a plastic container.

I pulled it out, and when I saw that it was an apple juice, I boohooed. It had been given to me at Roswell when I was admitted. Kenya must have put it in my purse before I was discharged.

That juice reminded me of where God brought me from, how He had set me free and how one moment in the presence of Jesus changed my life.

At the kitchen table, I told everyone, from here on out, "If I see apple juice, I'll cry."

Everybody laughed.

IT WASN'T FUNNY THEN

The apple juice story makes me laugh now, but it wasn't funny then. It sucks me into a time warp that puts me back in a terribly uncomfortable position.

In the wee hours of the morning, with the force of a firefighter's hose, my body violently spouted out the solution I needed to keep down in order to have a procedure done a few hours later. I was shocked. It was not supposed to happen like this; I mean, I was expecting to release what was inside, but not orally.

I had been expressly warned that, if my body did the exact thing it was doing, I was in trouble. It was a sign that I needed medical attention quickly.

Before things went haywire at approximately 2 am, for two days, I had been prepping for that colonoscopy I told you about. Specialists didn't like that I couldn't move my bowels despite being placed on the strongest laxatives they could prescribe.

On my X-rays, my specialist had identified an obstruction in my small intestine, and to figure out what was blocking me up, I needed to have a colonoscopy done. Once inside, they could take samples of the tissue in case there was a malignancy hidden there.

The process of getting my colon cleaned out wasn't supposed to be that big of a deal. My mother, who'd suffered with ulcerative colitis and had multiple colonoscopies without incident, said it was easy. Her advice was simple: "When they give you that solution to drink, it's very strong, so stay near the toilet." That sounded easy enough.

I thanked her for the tips and looked forward to releasing backed up wastes, since my body had not been able to expel toxins on its own. I was sick of the discomfort severe constipation caused. I was in constant pain; both my abdomen and my lower ribs on the left side ached. The first time I went to the ER, they told me, "We have never seen anyone with this much stool inside them."

During my colonoscopy prep, I thought, *Finally, I'll be able to get relief.* I was on a diet of clear liquids and laxatives. Day one went pretty well; day two is a different story entirely. I was required to chug a gallon of this disgusting, salty, weird-tasting fluid, reported to be the most-powerful-on-the-planet laxative. And that's when stuff got crazy.

THIS IS WHAT WE WERE WORRIED ABOUT

Although I didn't like the taste of the special drink, it's not that easy to activate my gag reflex, so I knocked it back like a pro; then, I waited for sweet relief. My life's goal had become to produce a healthy bowel movement.

My expectations were in the toilet—literally.

After guzzling, I waited with no results, until it was time to take another swill of the yucky stuff. And again, nothing happened. The more I chugged, the more uncomfortable I became.

My supposedly super-powerful bowel-cleansing drink, designed to purify me, wasn't working. My belly was full. Nothing passed, but time. Not even gas. Everything was trapped and I was miserable. A couple of hours later and I was doubled over in pain, trembling and sweating profusely.

It felt like my heart would pulsate out of my chest, and I was on the verge of losing consciousness. That's when the projectile vomiting happened. Kenya hurriedly placed a call to my medical team at Roswell.

The on-call doctor told him, "This is what we were worried about. This response is being caused by the obstruction and extreme narrowing in her small intestine."

When specialists get worried, there's a serious problem. That's when Kenya and I first learned exactly how concerned the medical team was about what they saw. I had to get to the emergency room without delay, but I could barely move without feeling as if I would explode.

Kenya had to help me into the minivan; I couldn't sit up, so he put pillows on the seat, laid me down, handed me a bag (because I was still feeling sick to my stomach), and hopped behind the wheel.

Each time he hit a bump, the impact punched me in the gut. It was, by far, one of the *longest* short road trips of my life. I moaned and groaned, silently praying for God to help me.

There were lots of people present when I arrived at the ER, hunched over, hoping not to lose the contents of my stomach in the waiting area. Of all nights, this would be the one where there had to be a long line of folks ahead of me. I was going to be sick again, so Kenya helped me to the restroom, where I stayed for about 45 minutes.

When I came out, I couldn't hold my head up, so I rested on Kenya, grunting and crying while he comforted me as best he could. I felt like I had the worst-ever-case of the stomach flu, times ten.

During the intake process, I held onto my plastic vomit bag the hospital staff gave me with quivering hands. I just wanted to be sedated; I'd do anything to make that feeling stop. Even thinking about it now makes me cringe. When they put in me in a room and monitored me, all my vital signs were going crazy, my bloodwork results were abnormal and alarming, and the medical team was puzzled.

THE ADVERSARY WAS UNDERCOVER

Even after hours of being there, they could not regulate me. They poked and prodded me, took scans and X-rays, drew more blood and drugged me.

When the lead physician came in to update me on my condition, I was told, "We took a look, and we see that your bowels have completely seized up, but we don't know why." She further expressed concern about my blood pressure, white and red blood cell count, and other troubling results. There was also lots of blood in my urine. That, too, was a mystery.

Not only was I in no condition to have my colonoscopy done, but I could not be discharged until whatever was driving my system nuts was under control. But how could doctors fight to control an enemy they could not recognize? The adversary was undercover, hiding. But eventually, God would both expose and expel him.

Hearing the perturbed MD go into detail about how negative my test results were, was sobering. At this time, I wasn't yet aware that my autoimmune diseases caused inflammation, which was responsible for locking up my bowels. But I knew enough to know I needed divine intervention. If God didn't rescue me, I was helpless and hopeless.

These are the events that led to me being admitted to Roswell, which I already told you about, so doctors could help me release all the wastes in my system. They tried to get me to drink apple juice to relieve me, but it wasn't strong enough. Eventually, they figured out how to get sporadic bowel breakthroughs. But the ultimate release I needed would have to come from the Balm in Gilead.

And He showed up at my healing service in a big way.

THEY LAID THEIR HANDS ON ME

My longtime friend and anointed psalmist, Serena Young, sang a song. I love her voice, her humility and her willingness to always be there when I need her. She's so giving that way. I can't remember what she was singing, though, because I was in a haze. After she finished, the intercessors, the 50 women, were called. They surrounded me and anointed me.

Evangelist Madge Whiskey, Minister Rhonda Smith, Mother Irene Wilson, and Cassandra Elliott were closest to me.

When they placed their hands on me, I was wondering, *Who told them where it hurt?* God had to be directing them, because everywhere they touched, was a place where the soreness and deeply embedded pain was most severe.

The power of God shot through my body. It felt like lightening, fire, and electricity hit me all at once. I was told I jerked violently, as if someone shocked me with a defibrillator. And suddenly, I heard this high-pitched scream. I wondered who it was.

Then I realized, it was me!

How could that be me?

I hadn't been able to sing or scream in months. Before I could process what was happening, I started moving and rocking. Some of the intercessors told me my legs were cold, like they didn't have any circulation in them, but when the power of God struck my lifeless limbs, my left leg kicked. My right one followed. Then, for the first time in months, I stood up, with no pain.

In the midst of a cloud of witnesses, I rose.

Evangelist Whiskey's fingers were interlocked with mine, and Kenya was right next to me. He told me he wasn't sure I was up under my own strength, and didn't want me to fall.

No, I wasn't up under my own strength, but under the power of God. It felt like someone had attached strings to my thighs and began pulling them up. It felt strange at first to lift my legs up so high. And then, I got this rush. I walked, then I ran, then I danced. Nobody was holding me. I wasn't winded. I wasn't sore.

I was healed.

By His stripes, I was—I am—healed.

I could not believe what had happened to me and I said as much into the microphone when Wynetta handed it to me. It was surreal, like something ripped right out of the pages of scripture. I sang that night in full voice, with no strain.

I preached that night. I shouted that night. The place erupted in praise. My mom and dad were rejoicing; Kenya and the children were crying and dancing before the Lord; family, friends, colleagues and co-laborers in the Kingdom were praising.

What a celebration it was!

I love looking back at photographs from the evening.

"Would it be okay if I donated my services that night," a gifted photographer named J' Marie Thomas warmly had offered in a conversation with Kenya prior to the healing service.

She captured priceless moments and I will treasure those images, and be grateful for her thoughtful generosity, forever.

GOD SPOKE DIRECTLY TO ME

After we celebrated, the intercessors prayed for those in attendance. Evangelist Wonda Core, an anointed vessel of God, released a powerful word that set our hearts ablaze. God gave her insight and revelation specific to that evening. It was so rich. I just love her spirit.

Then my dear sister-in-law, Bertha, the main speaker for the evening—who, along with the other ladies, had been fasting, praying and laying before the Lord leading up to that service—got the microphone.

When God told me she was the one anointed to bring forth the word that night, she was hesitant.

Lady B, as I like to call her, doesn't like the limelight and will happily work for the Kingdom in the shadows, but God called her for that hour.

And to think, she almost declined to speak because the Lord had already performed the miracle.

But He had something to say through her.

When Lady B finally agreed to release what He had given her, God spoke directly to me. It was like He had opened up everything I'd been through to her and used her mouth to say things only I could testify to as the truth.

She planted seeds of encouragement. She watered those dry places in me.

While there were others there in the sanctuary, I knew, the very God of Heaven was talking specifically to me.

IT WAS CONFIRMED

After that night, I went back to the doctor to be retested, and it was confirmed. I am whole. There are no traces of the diseases I had before my prayer service. God even disproved what the specialists told me about the damage that had been done to my joints and bones. They said it could not be reversed; but you know what God did? He reversed it. There are no traceable signs of erosion on any of my scans. My joints and bones are perfectly healthy.

God did it: suddenly; completely; in minutes; publicly. He did it for His glory.

I don't take any more medicines; no pain killers, no therapy. I have no limitations, no challenges, no explanation except, *God did it*.

In case you need a reminder, He is yet supernaturally intervening and disrupting natural cause-and-effect scenarios. He is flexing His dominion, authority and power, creating outcomes deemed impossible by human standards.

As much as I believe in the healing power of Jesus Christ and His ability to transform lives in an instant, I did not expect to be miraculously healed of two incurable autoimmune diseases in the way He chose to do it.

But I'm glad He did it.

REFLECTIONS

After I went back to my hotel room after my prayer service, you know what I did?

I raced the Hobbs children.

We tore through the hallways of the Sheraton, laughing and playing like schoolchildren on a playground. They hadn't seen their mom run or laugh like that in so long. I beat all of them, though I suspect they let me win.

When I got back into the room, one of the coolest things *ever* happened: I needed to move my bowels.

That may be kind of yucky, but it was God's way of saying, *Dianna, the work is completed. All of it.*

Now that I see the full picture of what happened to me from a different vantage point, from a position of wholeness, my perspective is clear. I had to go through all of that for the sake of the ministry. Others need to know what God is yet able to do.

I'm not jaded anymore; I am no longer blinded by pain, frustration, disillusionment and confusion. I don't have any regrets. I don't harbor any resentment about it. I know God allowed it to advance the work of the Kingdom.

These days, the sun is shining in the cloudless blue sky, and I can see clearly now that the rain is gone. Every day that I wake up and breathe in the fresh air, I am newly awed. When my feet hit the floor, I have no pain. I am still running, jumping and leaping to this day.

God has shown forth His goodness in my life in too many ways to count. I'll never be able to express to God, or to others I tell about His works, the magnitude of gratitude I feel in my heart.

Suffice it to say, I am overwhelmed.

ALL I KNOW

I don't know why He loves me. I don't know why He is gracious to me. Howbeit, there is something I *do* know.

There is a video of me on the Internet that captures the moments following my miraculous healing on the evening of March 26th. I have watched it many times over and wept. In the footage recorded and published by my brother, Bishop Joseph Brinson, Jr., I tell the congregation that I feel like the blind man healed by Jesus in John 9.

"All I know is I was blind, but now I see."

This is what the receiver of this incredible biblical miracle said after Jesus healed him by spitting in the dirt, making clay, rubbing it on his eyes, and commanding him to wash in the pool of Siloam.

I feel the same way *he* did.

All I know is, I *was* sick, and now I'm well.

All I know is, God did it!

A prayer for you: *God, please do it for them. Heal them, deliver them, and make a way. Water their dry places and bring liberty where they are bound.*

Answer their petitions; whatever their need or specific circumstance is. I am not in their shoes and don't know their predicament, but You do. I ask that You do a new thing in them. Turn things around for the better.

Loose them from any affliction and every infirmity. In Matthew 21:22 NLT, Your word tells us, "You can pray for anything, and if you have faith, you will receive it."

As they exercise their faith, I pray that You turn their test into a testimony of Your awesome power. Display through their life that there is no failure in You.

Just as You worked a miracle for me, do it for them. I believe they shall have it, according to Your will, and it is done.

In Jesus' name, Amen.

GET MORE INSPIRATION

To read Dianna's blog and hear her podcast, which are packed with uplifting, biblically sound inspiration, visit www.diannahobbs.com.

DIANNA HOBBS is the award-winning founder of Empowering Everyday Women Ministries, Inc., a non-profit organization that provides tools and resources to help women of faith grow stronger. She is the writer of "Your Daily Cup of Inspiration," named one of America's Top 100 blogs for women of faith by Women's Bible Café™. Her podcast and web publication, EEW Online, reaches a subscriber base of more than 250,000. Dianna and her husband Kenya, and the couple's four children, reside in Upstate New York.

Made in the USA
Middletown, DE
11 April 2018